Eviction Notice

Haley C. Horn

Eviction Notice

Life After Saying Goodbye To Your Uterus

Haley C. Horn

© 2025 Haley C. Horn

All rights reserved. No part of this publication may be reproduced, distributed, or transmitted in any form or by any means, including photocopying, recording, or other electronic or mechanical methods, without the prior written permission of the publisher, except in the case of brief quotations embodied in critical reviews and certain other noncommercial uses permitted by copyright law.

Printed in the United States of America

First Printing, March 2025.

Haley C. Horn
About the Book

Eviction Notice: Life After Saying Goodbye To Your Uterus is more than just a guide — it's a compassionate companion for women facing one of life's most profound crossroads. Whether your hysterectomy is planned, unexpected, or somewhere in between, this book speaks directly to your heart, your fears, and your hopes.

In a world where conversations about female health too often happen behind closed doors, this book opens the door wide. It meets you in the quiet moments of worry, the sleepless nights filled with unanswered questions, and the fragile space where grief and relief sometimes coexist.

Written by someone who has stood exactly where you are — staring down surgery, wondering what comes after — this book offers more than facts. It offers wisdom. It offers sisterhood. It offers a steady hand on your shoulder.

With warmth and honesty, you'll find:
- Clear, non-judgmental explanations of what hysterectomy really means — physically, emotionally, and intimately.
- Gentle preparation for what happens before, during, and after surgery — including the hard-to-ask questions no one else is talking about.
- Practical tools for healing your body and spirit, from pelvic floor health to coping with identity shifts.

Haley C. Horn

- Stories and reflections from others who have walked this path, reminding you that you are never alone in this experience.

This is not just a book about surgery. It's a book about reclaiming your power, redefining your femininity, and gently walking forward into a life that is still full, still vibrant, and still entirely yours — scar and all.

Haley C. Horn

Contents

About the Book	**4**
Preface	**8**
Part 1: Deciding on Surgery	**14**
Fibroids — What They Are, Where They Hide, and How They Affect You	14
NON-SURGICAL TREATMENTS FOR FIBROIDS: EXPLORING YOUR OPTIONS	19
REMOVING FIBROIDS: SURGICAL SOLUTIONS AND THEIR IMPLICATIONS	23
UTERINE PROLAPSE: UNDERSTANDING YOUR OPTIONS	28
PAIN AND ABNORMAL BLEEDING: WHEN TO BE CONCERNED	33
PRECANCEROUS CONDITIONS AND CANCER: MAKING INFORMED DECISIONS	39
PART 2: THE HYSTERECTOMY EXPERIENCE	**46**
Abdominal Hysterectomy	46
Vaginal Hysterectomy & Urinary Incontinence	50
Laparoscopic & Robotic-Assisted Hysterectomy	53
Hysterectomy Before Children: Navigating a Difficult Decision	58
Time-Sensitive Decisions: Planning Before Surgery	73
Talking to Your Doctor: Being Your Own Best Advocate	87
Choosing a Surgeon: Finding the Right Fit for You	93
Anesthesia and You: Understanding Your Options and Feeling Safe	97
Preparing for Surgery: Setting Yourself Up for a Smoother Recovery	101
The Day of Surgery — What Really Happens	106
The Operating Room — What Happens Once You're Inside	111
Part 3: Returning to Movement and Life After Surgery	**115**

Recovery Timeline 121
Understanding Your Post-Hysterectomy Body 126
Part 4: Life After Hysterectomy **133**
Hormone Replacement Therapy After Hysterectomy 133
SEXUALITY AND INTIMACY AFTER HYSTERECTOMY 138
Pelvic Floor Health: The Unsung Hero of Recovery 145
Glossary of Terms 151

Haley C. Horn

Preface

If you're holding this book right now, I know something about you already — you're standing at the edge of a life-changing moment.

You may have just been told you need a hysterectomy. Maybe you've suspected it for a while. Maybe you're searching late at night, looking for answers no one around you seems to have. Maybe you're trying to steady yourself, wondering how to make peace with a word that feels heavy and unfamiliar.

I know this moment. I've lived this moment. And you don't have to face it alone.

When I was told I needed a hysterectomy — before I had children, before I was ready — I felt like the world shifted under my feet. I scoured bookstores, online forums, and doctor's offices, searching for guidance that didn't just tell me the medical facts, but actually spoke to me, as a woman, as a person grieving, hoping, fearing, and yet somehow, still moving forward.

I couldn't find the book I needed then. So, I wrote it for you now.

This book is here to help you navigate what's ahead — the decisions, the emotions, the physical changes, the

Haley C. Horn
unexpected losses, and the surprising joys. You'll find practical information, but also gentle reassurance, the kind you might expect from a big sister or a dear friend who's been through it herself.

Whether you are terrified, numb, curious, or quietly strong, this book will sit beside you, not as a textbook, but as a companion.

You are allowed to feel what you feel. You are allowed to grieve, to hope, to rage, to heal — and you will.

My hope is simple: that you close this book knowing you are still whole, still powerful, and still deserving of a full, vibrant life — scar and all.

Haley C. Horn

Understanding Your Reproductive System, Myths, and Real Numbers — Getting the Full Picture

I remember sitting in that sterile doctor's office, staring at diagrams, trying hard to make sense of what was happening inside me. I realized quickly — understanding my own body wasn't just helpful, it was empowering. The more I learned, the less fear had power over me.

Your Reproductive System — More Than Just "Organs"

The female reproductive system is not just a set of parts, it's a beautifully interconnected system. Think of it like a well-rehearsed orchestra — each part playing its role, in harmony.

At the center is the uterus, often called the womb. It's shaped like an upside-down pear and sits low in your abdomen, protected by your pelvic bones. It's not just for pregnancy — it's a muscular powerhouse involved in your cycle, overall health, and even your posture. I never realized how much it was doing behind the scenes until my doctor walked me through it.

Attached to the uterus is the cervix, the narrow "neck" that connects the uterus to the vagina. It's like a flexible door — letting menstrual flow out, sperm in, and if you've ever given birth, you know it has an impressive ability to stretch when needed.

Next, there are the fallopian tubes, extending from either side of your uterus like tiny arms. They don't just sit there — they actively help guide eggs from your ovaries into the uterus. Your ovaries are two almond-sized glands that play a starring role. They produce estrogen and progesterone — the hormones that regulate your cycle, protect your bones, affect your mood, and even influence heart health.

This is why your doctor will talk carefully about whether or not your ovaries should be removed during surgery. It's not just about fertility — it's about your body's long-term balance.

Myth vs. Reality — Let's Get Real

During my pre-surgery deep dive, I ran into so many scary myths online. I get it — when you're anxious, the internet can be both your best friend and worst enemy. Let's clear up a few common ones:

`Myth #1: You'll go straight into menopause after a hysterectomy.`

Not always. Menopause only happens immediately if your ovaries are removed. If they stay put, your hormones keep flowing like before. I can still remember the relief I felt when I learned I could keep my ovaries.

`Myth #2: Your sex life is over.`

Haley C. Horn

Honestly? Many women say it improves — sometimes a lot. No more pain from fibroids, heavy bleeding, or constant discomfort. The vagina's structure doesn't disappear, and as long as healing goes well, intimacy remains — and can even become more enjoyable.

Myth #3: You'll have a weird "gap" or change shape.

Nope. Your pelvic floor and other tissues naturally shift and adjust after surgery, but it doesn't change how you look on the outside. I used to worry about this, and looking back, it was one of the silliest fears — but a real one for me at the time.

Myth #4: Recovery takes forever.

Not true for everyone. Yes, full healing inside takes about 6–8 weeks, but many women are back to light activities within a few weeks. I was back at work by week three — cautiously, but feeling stronger every day.

The Numbers — Why They Matter to You

- About 600,000 hysterectomies are performed each year in the U.S. — you are definitely not alone.
- By age 60, roughly 1 in 3 American women will have had a hysterectomy.
- The average age is around 42, but it varies.
- Around 90% of surgeries are for non-cancerous conditions like fibroids, endometriosis, or heavy bleeding.

Haley C. Horn

- More than 60% today are performed using minimally invasive techniques, helping reduce recovery time.

I found comfort in these numbers. I wasn't the only one going through this. Understanding the science and the statistics gave me a clearer mind when it came time to make my own decisions.

The more you understand your body, the more power you have when it comes to making health choices. When I faced the possibility of surgery, learning about my reproductive system was like turning on a light in a dark room — suddenly, I could see the path ahead.

Haley C. Horn

Part 1: Deciding on Surgery

Fibroids — What They Are, Where They Hide, and How They Affect You

The first time I saw my ultrasound, I felt frozen. What was supposed to be a routine check-up revealed not just one, but multiple growths. The largest? About the size of a lemon. Like many women, I had heard of fibroids before, but I hadn't given them much thought. Now, faced with them firsthand, I realized how little I truly knew.

Since then, I've met many women with similar stories. Some had tiny fibroids causing chaos, others had large ones hiding quietly. In this section, I want to help you make sense of what fibroids really are, where they grow, and how they can affect your body and life — just like someone did for me when I needed it most.

Types and Locations of Fibroids — Where They Show Up Matters

Fibroids (also called leiomyomas or myomas) are non-cancerous tumors that form inside or around the uterus. Think of your uterus as a small house, and fibroids as uninvited guests — where they show up influences the trouble they cause.

Subserosal Fibroids

These grow on the outside of the uterus, like a bump pushing outward. Depending on where they press, they can make you feel constant pressure or discomfort. Maria, a woman I met at a support group, told me how hers pressed on her bladder so much that she was afraid to leave the house without knowing where every restroom was.

Intramural Fibroids

These are the most common. They grow within the uterine wall, making the uterus feel swollen or heavy. They can cause heavy bleeding, pressure, and sometimes even back pain. Many women describe it as walking around with a "weighted ball" inside.

Submucosal Fibroids

These form just beneath the uterine lining and protrude into the uterine cavity. Even small ones can cause extreme bleeding. Sarah, a teacher I spoke with, had a submucosal fibroid the size of a grape — small, right? But it led to such severe blood loss that she became anemic and struggled with daily fatigue.

Pedunculated Fibroids

These are attached by a thin stalk, either inside or outside the uterus, almost like cherries on stems. They may twist unexpectedly, causing sudden sharp pain.

Common Symptoms — But Not Always Obvious

One of the trickiest things about fibroids is that some women have zero symptoms, while others experience life-altering challenges. Here are common signs:

- **Heavy menstrual bleeding**
  Long, heavy periods, clots, and even bleeding between periods.
  I remember carrying extra clothes in my work bag just in case. I thought I was being overly cautious until I realized how many other women do the same.

- **Pressure and pain**
  Lower back pain, pelvic pressure, bloating, constipation, frequent urination, and difficulty emptying the bladder.

- **Reproductive challenges**
  Fibroids can sometimes interfere with conception, cause miscarriages, complicate pregnancies, or make intimacy painful.

How Fibroids Impact Your Life — More Than Just Physical

Haley C. Horn

What surprised me most was how fibroids can quietly shape every corner of your life — not just your body.

- Work
 Missed days due to exhaustion or pain. Skipping important meetings out of fear of unexpected bleeding.

- Social life
 Avoiding outings because you don't trust your body. Cancelling plans last minute because of pain or bleeding.

- Relationships
 Strain from painful intercourse, anxiety about fertility, or the emotional drain of feeling like you're "not yourself."

- Mental health
 Worry, depression, frustration — sometimes it's not just the physical symptoms that hurt, but the constant reminder that you're not in control.

Lisa, a 41-year-old executive, told me, "I was up for a major promotion, but I lived in fear of bleeding through my clothes during presentations. It wasn't just inconvenient — it changed the way I showed up for myself."

How Doctors Diagnose Fibroids — What to Expect

I didn't realize there were so many tests available until I was going through them myself. Knowing what's coming can make things less intimidating:

Haley C. Horn

Pelvic Exam
Your doctor may feel your uterus to check for enlargement or irregularities, but smaller fibroids often go unnoticed without imaging.

Ultrasound
This is the most common first step.
- Transabdominal — moves over your abdomen.
- Transvaginal — uses a wand-shaped probe for a clearer view.

My fibroid journey started here — and honestly, seeing the ultrasound made everything more real.

MRI
Provides detailed images, helpful when your doctor is planning surgery or distinguishing fibroids from other conditions.

Sonohysterography
A specialized ultrasound where saline expands the uterus, making submucosal fibroids easier to spot.

Hysteroscopy
A tiny camera inserted through the cervix gives a direct look inside the uterus. In some cases, your doctor can treat small fibroids during this procedure.

Endometrial Biopsy
Not to detect fibroids directly, but sometimes used to rule out other causes of irregular bleeding

Reflection Moment

Haley C. Horn

> Before you rush to decisions, take a breath.
> - How are your symptoms affecting your day-to-day life?
> - Are you adjusting your work, relationships, or social life because of fibroids?
> - What does quality of life mean to you right now?

This is about more than just test results — it's about your comfort, confidence, and ability to show up fully in your life.

NON-SURGICAL TREATMENTS FOR FIBROIDS: EXPLORING YOUR OPTIONS

Before I underwent my hysterectomy, I spent nearly two years navigating the maze of non-surgical treatments, hoping to avoid surgery altogether. Like many women, I wished for relief without the thought of an operating room. While these therapies didn't give me lasting results, they do offer hope and solutions for many others. Let's explore the full range of non-surgical options available, their benefits, and their limitations.

Medical and Hormonal Therapy

Hormonal Birth Control Options

Haley C. Horn

Often the first line of defense, hormonal treatments help control symptoms such as heavy bleeding and painful periods. These include:
- Combined oral contraceptives
- Hormonal IUDs (e.g., Mirena)
- Progesterone-only pills
- Injectable contraceptives

I personally tried a hormonal IUD, which did help reduce my bleeding temporarily, though it didn't shrink my fibroids. Janet, a 37-year-old nurse I met during treatment, found complete relief through her IUD. It's important to know that what works beautifully for one woman might only partially help another.

GnRH Agonists (Gonadotropin-Releasing Hormone)
These medications temporarily shrink fibroids by putting your body into a state similar to menopause.
- Common brands include Lupron, Synarel, and Zoladex.
- Treatment is usually short-term (3–6 months) and often used to shrink fibroids before surgery.

Side effects may include hot flashes, mood changes, and potential bone loss if used too long. As my gynecologist once told me, "It's like pressing pause on your hormones — but not forever." Once the medication is stopped, fibroids may regrow.

Non-Hormonal Treatments
These don't shrink fibroids but help control symptoms:
- Tranexamic Acid (Lysteda) to reduce heavy bleeding.
- NSAIDs for pain relief.
- Iron supplements to combat anemia.

Eviction Notice

Haley C. Horn

Uterine Artery Embolization (UAE)

The UAE has changed the game for many women. This minimally invasive procedure blocks the blood supply feeding fibroids, causing them to shrink.
- Performed by an interventional radiologist.
- A small incision is made, and particles are injected to block targeted blood vessels.
- Recovery is typically 1–2 weeks.

Sarah, who I interviewed years after her UAE, was still thrilled with her choice and living symptom-free. However, the UAE is not ideal for everyone. Large fibroids, certain locations, and future pregnancy plans may influence if this is right for you.

MRI-Guided Focused Ultrasound (MRgFUS)

MRgFUS is a high-tech, non-invasive therapy that uses focused ultrasound waves (guided by MRI) to destroy fibroid tissue without harming healthy tissue.
- Outpatient procedure (no incisions).
- Recovery is often just a few days.
- Best for women with smaller, well-located fibroids.

Rebecca, a 42-year-old athlete, chose MRgFUS to minimize downtime and was able to resume training shortly after. However, this option may not be widely available, and insurance coverage can vary.

Haley C. Horn

Complementary and Alternative Therapies

Many women also turn to natural or alternative remedies:
- Dietary Adjustments: Emphasize anti-inflammatory foods, leafy greens, limit processed food, caffeine, and alcohol.
- Supplements: Vitamin D, turmeric, green tea extract, fish oil, and iron (if anemic).
- Mind-Body Therapies: Acupuncture, massage, and stress-reduction practices may help with pain and emotional well-being.

I incorporated many of these during my journey, and while they didn't shrink my fibroids, they helped me cope physically and emotionally.

Always consult your healthcare provider before starting supplements or alternative treatments to avoid interference with medications or causing unintended effects.

Knowing When to Consider Surgery

Haley C. Horn

It's important to recognize when non-surgical treatments are no longer enough. Some signs that surgery may be the next step include:
- Severe bleeding despite treatment.
- Uncontrolled pain or pressure.
- Chronic anemia.
- Daily life and emotional well-being are significantly affected.
- Fibroids keep growing despite therapy.
- Repeated treatment failures.

For me, the hardest realization was that I was spending more time managing symptoms than enjoying life. Once I accepted that, I could clearly consider surgery as a next step — not as defeat, but as self-care.

> **Pause & Reflect**
> - Which treatments from this section have you tried, or are you considering?
> - How are your current symptoms affecting your quality of life?

Haley C. Horn

- Are you feeling empowered to have a deeper conversation with your doctor about your options?

Jot your thoughts down, or simply reflect on them quietly.

REMOVING FIBROIDS: SURGICAL SOLUTIONS AND THEIR IMPLICATIONS

When I first sat in my doctor's office facing the possibility of fibroid removal, I remember feeling overwhelmed by the sheer variety of surgical options. The medical terms, diagrams, and risks seemed like a lot to absorb. Now, looking back, I see how essential it was to understand that each surgery comes with its own set of advantages and challenges. In this chapter, I want to help you navigate these choices so you can make the one that fits your body, goals, and life.

Myomectomy: Removing the Fibroids, Preserving the Uterus

Myomectomy refers to the surgical removal of fibroids while keeping the uterus intact — a vital consideration if you wish to maintain fertility or simply want to avoid hysterectomy.

Types of Myomectomy:

1. Abdominal Myomectomy (Open Surgery)

- Performed through a larger incision (similar to a C-section).
- Best for: Multiple, large, or deeply embedded fibroids.
- Recovery: 4–6 weeks, with a hospital stay of 2–3 days.

My colleague Elena chose this route. She had several large fibroids but still wanted the option to have children. "The recovery wasn't easy," she confided, "but keeping my uterus was worth every step."

2. Laparoscopic Myomectomy
   - Performed using several small incisions and specialized instruments.
   - Best for: Smaller or fewer fibroids.
   - Recovery: 2–3 weeks, often as an outpatient or with a short hospital stay.
   - Requires a highly skilled surgeon for optimal results.

3. Hysteroscopic Myomectomy
   - Performed vaginally without external incisions.
   - Best for: Fibroids located inside the uterine cavity (submucosal).
   - Recovery: Fast — usually 2–3 days.
   - Limitation: Only suitable for certain fibroids, and some women may need more than one procedure.

4. Robot-Assisted Myomectomy
   - Uses robotic technology for enhanced precision.
   - Similar to laparoscopic but offers better visualization and dexterity.
   - Often more expensive and less available but increasingly popular in specialized centers.

Haley C. Horn

> **Reflection Box:**
> Which of these options aligns with your current health goals?
> - Is fertility preservation important to you?
> - Are you comfortable with a longer recovery for potentially better long-term results?

Risks Associated with Myomectomy

Surgery always carries risks, and understanding them can help you make an informed choice:

- Bleeding, which may rarely require a transfusion.
- Infection or injury to nearby organs.
- Adhesions (internal scar tissue) that can cause pelvic pain or fertility issues.
- Recurrence, as fibroids may grow back over time.
- Impact on future pregnancies, depending on how much of the uterus was altered.

I appreciated that my doctor didn't sugarcoat these risks. Janet, a fellow patient, told me, "My first myomectomy gave me great relief, but new fibroids came back within three years. Knowing this ahead of time helped me prepare mentally."

Recovery varies depending on the type of surgery and your body's healing capacity.

When Might Hysterectomy Be the Better Option?

After two myomectomies and multiple fibroid recurrences, I personally arrived at this crossroad. Here are common situations where a hysterectomy may be the recommended path:

Medical Considerations:
- Multiple or very large fibroids.
- Persistent bleeding and anemia.
- Prior unsuccessful surgeries.
- Approaching menopause.
- Other uterine conditions like adenomyosis.

Personal Considerations:
- Family building is complete.
- Seeking a definitive solution.
- Repeated surgical expenses are unsustainable.
- Symptoms severely reduce quality of life.

For me, it came down to this: after years of treatments, ongoing discomfort, and missed life moments, I needed a lasting solution. Choosing hysterectomy wasn't giving up — it was taking control.

Ask Yourself:
```
1. Am I ready to part with my uterus if it
improves my health and quality of life?
2. Am I emotionally and physically prepared for
either choice?
```

3. Do I have the support I need during the recovery phase?

Pro Tip:
Dr. Martinez, a gynecologic surgeon I consulted, said it perfectly: "The best surgical option isn't just about fibroids; it's about the woman sitting in front of me, her goals, her fears, and her life."

Choosing between myomectomy and hysterectomy is not just a medical decision — it's deeply personal. There is no wrong choice, only what is right for you at this stage of your life.

UTERINE PROLAPSE: UNDERSTANDING YOUR OPTIONS

When Jane, a 55-year-old yoga teacher, first noticed a bulge in her vaginal area, she brushed it off as part of getting older. Only when simple tasks like walking, standing, and exercising became uncomfortable did she finally seek medical advice. Her story is one I've heard repeatedly — uterine prolapse often creeps up slowly but can end up significantly affecting daily life. The good news is, there are many ways to manage it.

Stages of Prolapse: Where Do You Stand?

Understanding prolapse stages helps you and your doctor choose the most appropriate treatment.

Stage 0 : Normal uterus position (No symptoms)

Stage 1 (Mild): Uterus drops slightly into the upper vagina (Often detected during routine checkups; may cause few or no symptoms)

Stage 2 (Moderate): Uterus descends near the vaginal opening (Noticeable pressure, heaviness, or discomfort)

Stage 3 (Advanced): Uterus partially protrudes beyond the vaginal opening (Symptoms interfere with daily life)

Stage 4 (Complete): Uterus fully protrudes outside the vaginal opening (Severe symptoms and urgent need for treatment)

Reflection Box:
```
- Do I know which stage I might be in?
- Have I had a proper pelvic exam to assess my
prolapse?
- How much does it currently affect my daily
activities?
```

Conservative Management: The First Line of Defense

Before considering surgery, many women find relief with conservative options.

Lifestyle Adjustments:

- Maintain a healthy weight.
- Avoid heavy lifting.
- Manage chronic cough or constipation.
- Quit smoking.

Pelvic Floor Therapy:
- Kegel exercises.
- Pelvic floor physical therapy with biofeedback.
- Core strengthening and breathing techniques.

Like Janet, who told me, "I was doubtful at first, but after three months of focused pelvic therapy, I saw real improvement," many women find that consistent effort pays off.

Pessary Use: A Non-Surgical Ally

Pessaries are silicone devices inserted into the vagina to support the uterus and vaginal walls.

Types of Pessaries:
- Ring (most common)
- Gellhorn
- Cube
- Donut
- Support pessaries (varies based on anatomy and severity)

Pessary Care:
- Regular removal and cleaning.
- Professional fitting and follow-up.
- Sometimes combined with vaginal estrogen to maintain vaginal tissue health.

Mary shared, "My pessary allowed me to continue hiking and teaching yoga. Once I got used to it, it became second nature."

Challenges:
Initial fitting, learning insertion/removal, dealing with discharge, and scheduling regular check-ups.

When Surgery Becomes the Best Choice

While many women manage prolapse without surgery, certain signs may indicate it's time to consider a more permanent solution:

Medical Indicators:
- Conservative options have failed.
- Pessary use is uncomfortable or ineffective.
- Prolapse is worsening.
- Symptoms now include ulcers, bleeding, bladder or bowel problems.

Quality of Life Indicators:
- Avoiding social and work activities.
- Painful or impossible sexual activity.
- Constant discomfort or distress.

Surgical Options for Uterine Prolapse

1. Vaginal Approach
- No external incisions.

- Shorter recovery.
- Ideal for certain prolapse types.

2. Abdominal Approach (Open or Laparoscopic)
- Longer-lasting results.
- Preferred in advanced or complex cases.
- May involve abdominal incisions or minimally invasive techniques.

3. Robotic-Assisted Surgery
- Minimally invasive.
- Quicker recovery.
- Requires specialized surgical expertise.

Reflection Box:
```
Am I ready for surgery, or is there more I want
to try first?
- Have I maximized all conservative options?
- How much is prolapse limiting my life?
```

Questions to Ask Your Doctor:
- What stage is my prolapse?
- Are there any non-surgical options left for me to try?
- Which surgical method suits my case best?
- What is the likely recovery time?
- What are the risks and benefits for me personally?
- Will my insurance cover the recommended treatment?

Dr. Thompson, a compassionate urogynecologist I met, explained, "Surgery is rarely the first step, but for many women, it restores the life they've been slowly losing. The key is timing — not too soon, but not too late."

Personal Advice:
Keep a journal of your symptoms. Record:
- Changes over time.
- How prolapse limits your daily life.
- Results of conservative treatments.

This simple habit will prepare you and your healthcare team to make clear, informed decisions — without the pressure of guessing.

PAIN AND ABNORMAL BLEEDING: WHEN TO BE CONCERNED

I remember sitting across from my gynecologist, struggling to describe what I was going through. "It's probably normal," I kept telling myself, even though I had missed work due to intense pain and bleeding. Like many women, I had unknowingly accepted what was actually a serious medical issue. Understanding the difference between normal and abnormal is crucial — and can be life-changing.

Understanding What's Normal — and What Isn't

Haley C. Horn

Normal Menstrual Patterns:
- Cycle length: 21–35 days
- Bleeding lasts: 3–7 days
- Flow: About 3–6 pads or tampons per day
- Mild to moderate cramping manageable with over-the-counter medications
- Predictable timing and tolerable mood shifts

Red Flags — Signs to Take Seriously:
- Soaking through a pad or tampon every hour
- Bleeding lasting longer than 7 days
- Passing blood clots larger than a quarter
- Bleeding between periods
- Bleeding after sex
- Bleeding after menopause

Sarah shared with me, "I thought heavy periods were just part of the package until my doctor told me that soaking an extra tampon every hour wasn't normal. That conversation changed my life."

Pain Patterns That Deserve Attention:

Typical Pain:
- Mild to moderate cramping during periods
- Relieved by OTC pain medication
- Does not disrupt daily life

Abnormal Pain:
- Severe cramps
- Pain throughout the entire cycle, not just during menstruation

- Pain that does not respond to medication
- Pain interfering with work, relationships, or daily routines
- Pain during sex
- Lower back, bladder, or bowel pain

Endometriosis & Adenomyosis: Silent Saboteurs

Endometriosis:

A common but often underdiagnosed condition where uterine-like tissue grows outside the uterus, sometimes even on other organs.

Common Symptoms:
- Severe menstrual pain
- Painful sex
- Bowel or bladder discomfort
- Fatigue
- Nausea
- Infertility concerns

Endometriosis affects 1 in 10 women and is frequently diagnosed only after years of unexplained suffering.

Adenomyosis:

Occurs when endometrial tissue grows into the muscular wall of the uterus, often causing uterine enlargement. More common in women over 40 and sometimes confused with fibroids.

Typical Symptoms:
- Heavy periods
- Severe cramps

Haley C. Horn

- Deep pelvic pain
- Painful intercourse
- May improve after menopause

> **Reflection Box:**
> ```
> Could I be experiencing endometriosis or
> adenomyosis?
> - Are my periods heavier or more painful than
> what is described as typical?
> - Do I have pain beyond just my menstrual
> cycle?
> ```

Lisa confided, "I planned everything — vacations, work events, even my wedding — around my cycle. I didn't realize how much control it had over my life."

When to Escalate Treatment

Starting with first-line options is common, but don't hesitate to seek more advanced care if needed.

First-Line Treatments:
- Over-the-counter pain relievers
- Heat therapy
- Birth control pills
- Lifestyle modifications (exercise, stress management, diet)

When to Consider More:
- Symptoms worsen

Haley C. Horn

- First-line therapies aren't enough
- You develop anemia
- Mental health is affected
- Life feels like it's revolving around pain or bleeding

Secondary Treatments:
- Hormonal IUDs
- Injectable contraceptives
- Prescription pain management
- Endometrial ablation
- GnRH agonists

Surgical Treatments:
- Laparoscopic excision of endometriosis
- Uterine artery embolization
- Myomectomy (if fibroids are involved)
- Hysterectomy

Making Treatment Decisions: Personal & Practical Factors

Questions to Guide You:
1. How severe are my symptoms?
2. Have I tried and documented conservative treatments?
3. How much is my daily life limited?
4. What are my fertility goals?
5. What can I afford? Will my insurance cover the options I need?

Helpful Tip:
Keep a journal of:
- Bleeding patterns

- Pain levels
- Missed activities or workdays
- Emotional strain
- Results of each treatment tried

Dr. Rodriguez, a pelvic pain specialist, wisely advised me, "Don't wait until pain controls your entire life. Early intervention opens more doors to relief."

When Hysterectomy Might Be the Right Step

While often a last resort, a hysterectomy can be life-changing for women facing:

- Chronic, uncontrollable pain and bleeding
- Failed conservative treatments
- Completed childbearing
- Multiple pelvic conditions at once
- Significant decline in quality of life

Personal Considerations:
- Age and health
- Fertility goals
- Support system
- Emotional readiness
- Finances and insurance coverage
- Recovery time available

Remember:
Pain and abnormal bleeding are not "just part of being a woman." They are valid, treatable medical conditions. The

next section will explore precancerous and cancerous conditions — where early detection is especially crucial.

PRECANCEROUS CONDITIONS AND CANCER: MAKING INFORMED DECISIONS

When I first read the word "precancerous" on my pathology report, it felt like the ground disappeared beneath me. The word cancer brings immediate fear — but understanding the spectrum of cellular changes, their risks, and treatment options empowers you to make informed, thoughtful decisions.

Decoding Your Pathology Report

Not all abnormal cells are cancerous. Many are precancerous or even benign. Understanding the terminology is the first step to calm and clarity.

- Normal: Cells look and behave as expected. No concerns
- Benign Changes: Non-cancerous changes. Often monitored without immediate treatment
- Precancerous: Cells show abnormal patterns but are not cancer yet. Treatment depends on severity.

- Carcinoma in Situ: Cancer cells are present but contained. They haven't spread yet
- Invasive Cancer: Cancer cells have spread beyond their original location. Immediate treatment needed

Grades of Precancerous Changes:

1. Mild Dysplasia (CIN 1)
- Often resolves naturally
- Close monitoring recommended
- Around 60% will revert to normal

2. Moderate Dysplasia (CIN 2)
- Intermediate risk
- Usually requires treatment
- Regular follow-up is key

3. Severe Dysplasia (CIN 3)
- High risk of progressing to cancer
- Prompt treatment advised

Dr. Chen once told me, "Think of precancerous changes like traffic lights — green for watchful waiting, yellow for caution and closer observation, and red for action."

Reflection Box:
What's my diagnosis?
- Has my doctor clearly explained the grade of my precancerous condition?

Haley C. Horn

- Am I clear on whether monitoring or immediate treatment is needed?

Should I Consider Genetic Testing?

Genetic testing is worth discussing if you:
- Have a strong family history of cancers
- Were diagnosed young
- Have relatives with multiple cancer types
- Belong to a high-risk ethnic group

The Process:
1. Genetic counseling
2. Risk assessment
3. Blood or saliva testing
4. Interpreting results with your healthcare team
5. Personalized treatment planning

Reflection Box:
Could genetic testing help me?
- Do I have a family history of cancer?
- Would knowing my genetic status affect my treatment decisions?

Urgency: When Is Immediate Action Needed?

When Immediate Treatment Is Recommended:
- CIN 2 or CIN 3 (moderate to severe dysplasia)
- Invasive cancer
- Symptoms worsening rapidly

Eviction Notice

Haley C. Horn
- High-risk genetic status

When Close Monitoring May Be Appropriate:
- CIN 1 or mild precancerous changes
- Stable condition
- No severe symptoms
- Reliable access to follow-up care

Dr. Thompson advises, "Act decisively when necessary, but don't rush into invasive treatment if conservative options are safe and effective."

Life Factors That Influence Timing:
- Fertility preservation
- Emotional readiness
- Insurance coverage
- Availability of a support system
- Work-life balance and caregiving duties

Reflection Box:
```
What is right for me?
- What is my personal tolerance for risk?
- Do I want to preserve fertility?
- How do I feel about balancing treatment
intensity with life impact?
```

Key Questions to Ask Your Doctor:
- What exactly does my pathology report say?
- What are all my treatment options?
- What is the success rate for each?
- How urgent is it to begin treatment?

Haley C. Horn

- What happens if I wait?
- How will this affect my fertility and hormones?
- Will insurance cover the recommended treatments?

Making Informed, Empowered Choices

It's natural to feel overwhelmed when hearing words like "precancerous" or "abnormal." But knowledge is power. Many precancerous conditions can be treated effectively, and you have options.

As Dr. Thompson often reminds his patients, "The goal is to treat enough to protect you without overtreating conditions that might resolve naturally."

PART 2: THE HYSTERECTOMY EXPERIENCE

Abdominal Hysterectomy

When my doctor first mentioned abdominal hysterectomy, all I could picture was a large incision, weeks of pain, and a long, lonely recovery. But learning the facts—and hearing real stories from women who had been through it—helped me see it for what it really is: a path to relief, healing, and sometimes, a whole new chapter.

The Classical Open Surgery

An abdominal hysterectomy is often called the traditional approach, and for good reason. It has been the go-to method when surgeons need full visibility and access to the pelvic organs.

Technique Basics:
- Involves a horizontal (bikini line) or vertical incision
- Gives the surgeon a clear, wide view of the pelvic area
- Allows direct handling of organs, helpful in complex cases
- Often chosen when minimally invasive options aren't safe

Haley C. Horn

Dr. Martinez once explained it to me simply: "Think of it like opening a book—you need full access to every page when the story is complicated."

Surgical Journey Step by Step

1. Preoperative Preparation
   - Bowel preparation (in some cases)
   - Fasting
   - Adjusting medications
   - Hospital admission
   - Meeting the anesthesia team

2. Surgery Day
   - General anesthesia
   - The incision (horizontal or vertical, depending on your case)
   - Careful removal of the uterus, and sometimes the ovaries or cervix
   - Closure of the layers of tissue and skin

When Is It the Right Choice?

While less common today thanks to laparoscopic options, abdominal hysterectomy is still the safest option for certain situations:

- Very large fibroids (Too big for laparoscopic instruments)
- Multiple prior surgeries (Scar tissue may complicate minimally invasive approaches)

Haley C. Horn

- Extensive adhesions (Abdominal entry gives better access)
- Cancer (Need for wide exposure and exploration)
- Complex anatomy (Congenital variations or unexpected findings)

Leah, a fellow patient, told me, "At first I was disappointed to need the traditional surgery. But knowing it was the safest route for my situation helped me trust the process and focus on recovery."

What to Expect in the Hospital

Before Surgery:
- Pre-op testing
- Meeting your surgical and anesthesia teams
- IV placement
- Going over last-minute questions

Surgery Day:
- 1 to 3-hour procedure
- 1 to 2 hours in recovery
- Beginning pain management
- Early gentle movement (yes, even the first day!)

Hospital Stay (Typically 2-4 Days):

- Day 1: Pain relief, first walk, clear liquids, catheter removal
- Day 2: Walking in hallways, advancing to solid foods, learning wound care |

- Day 3-4: Independent walking, preparing for discharge, getting home care instructions

The Recovery Timeline (Realistic, Not Sugar-Coated)

- Week 1: Lots of rest, pain meds, help needed, caring for your incision
- Weeks 2-3: Starting light movement, less medication, still limited activity
- Weeks 4-6: Returning to light work (if you feel ready), more mobility, emotional ups and downs normal
- Weeks 6-12: Gradually returning to regular life, sexual activity cleared, full healing continues

Dr. Martinez told me, "Everyone recovers at their own pace. Don't rush it."

Tips I Give to Every Woman Facing This:

- Set up your home for comfort before surgery
- Don't try to be a superhero—get help
- Have entertainment ready (TV shows, books, crafts)
- Be gentle with yourself emotionally
- Expect ups and downs
- Listen to your body

Haley C. Horn

Vaginal Hysterectomy & Urinary Incontinence

When I first heard about the vaginal hysterectomy, I imagined something complicated, mysterious, and possibly riskier. What I didn't expect was that many women describe it as the "quieter," easier surgery—the one with an invisible scar and, often, an unexpectedly smooth recovery. After talking with dozens of patients and surgeons, I realized that this technique holds a powerful but underappreciated place in women's healthcare.

Why Choose the Vaginal Approach?

Vaginal hysterectomy isn't just about removing the uterus—it's about doing it in a way that often feels more gentle on the body.

Surgical Advantages:
- No external incisions
- Shorter hospital stay (1-2 days)
- Less pain after surgery
- Quicker return to normal activities
- Lower complication rates
- Better cosmetic outcome—no visible scar

Dr. Williams, a urogynecologist, told me, "Think of it as using a backdoor shortcut—it's often the most direct and least disruptive path."

Who Is It Right For?

Not every woman is a candidate for vaginal hysterectomy, but for those who are, it can be life-changing.

Ideal Candidates:
- Smaller or moderately sized uterus
- Mobile uterus
- Limited history of abdominal surgeries
- No need for extensive exploration
- Good pelvic support

Maria shared:
"I was amazed that such a major surgery could be done without any visible scars. Three weeks later, I was back at work, and nobody could tell I'd even had surgery."

The Power of Combined Procedures

One of the hidden benefits of the vaginal approach is that surgeons often combine it with pelvic floor repairs or urinary incontinence treatments—addressing multiple problems in one operation.

Common Add-Ons:
1. Stress Urinary Incontinence Treatments:
   - Sling procedures

Haley C. Horn
- Bladder neck suspension
- Urethral bulking agents

2. Pelvic Organ Prolapse Repairs:
   - Anterior repair (bladder support)
   - Posterior repair (rectal wall support)
   - Vaginal vault suspension
   - Ligament reinforcement

Sarah explained it best:
"Having my prolapse and incontinence fixed during my hysterectomy was like getting a complete pelvic renovation. One surgery, multiple solutions."

Recovery: Faster, Smoother, Gentler

Compared to abdominal surgery, vaginal hysterectomy often offers a noticeably smoother recovery.

- Hospital Stay: 1-2 days, early mobility, light meals quickly
- First Week: Less pain medication, more independence, light walking
- Weeks 2-4: More activity, resume light chores, possible return to driving
- Weeks 4-6: Rebuilding stamina, better sleep, gradual emotional recovery

Special Tips:
- Pelvic rest (no intercourse or heavy lifting) for 6-8 weeks
- Manage vaginal discharge
- Pelvic floor exercises are key

Haley C. Horn

- Regular follow-ups to monitor healing

Dr. Chen's advice to patients:
"Let your body be your guide—move gently, rest fully, and trust the healing process."

Lisa wrote in her recovery journal:
"By week three, I was taking short walks. By week six, I felt almost normal. The vaginal approach made recovery so much smoother than I expected."

Long-Term Outcomes

- Excellent patient satisfaction
- Long-lasting results
- Restored pelvic function
- Improved sexual health
- Relief from urinary symptoms
- Confidence in daily life restored

Vaginal hysterectomy is not suitable for everyone—but when it is, it often delivers more than just symptom relief. It can address urinary incontinence, prolapse, and pelvic pain, all while offering a smoother recovery.

Remember:
- Scars aren't the only thing invisible—so is the quiet strength you'll gain.
- Your surgical plan should be as unique as you are.
- Combined procedures can give you your life back.

Haley C. Horn
Laparoscopic & Robotic-Assisted Hysterectomy

When I first learned about laparoscopic and robotic-assisted hysterectomies, I was skeptical—could technology really make such a big difference? After speaking with patients, surgeons, and witnessing these procedures myself, I can confidently say: these modern approaches have redefined how we approach hysterectomy.

Technology at Work: The Tools Behind the Surgery

These aren't just fancy gadgets—they are precision instruments designed to make surgery less invasive and recovery faster.

Laparoscopic Equipment:
- High-definition cameras
- Specialized long instruments
- Carbon dioxide inflation to create space
- Energy sealing tools
- Real-time imaging systems

Dr. Roberts explained it best:
"Laparoscopic surgery is like doing intricate work through keyholes. We see everything magnified on HD screens, which lets us operate with incredible precision."

Robotic-Assisted Surgery:

- Surgeon console (the brain)
- Robotic arms (the hands)
- 3D vision system
- Wristed instruments with full range of motion
- Tremor filtration technology

Unlike what some patients imagine, robots don't operate independently. Surgeons fully control every movement through a console, combining the robot's precision with human judgment.

Benefits of Minimally Invasive Hysterectomy

For many, these modern approaches bring real advantages:

Why Patients Love It:
- Tiny incisions (just a few centimeters)
- Minimal scarring
- Less postoperative pain
- Reduced infection risk
- Shorter hospital stay
- Quicker return to daily life

Why Surgeons Love It:
- 10x magnification
- Crystal-clear 3D imaging
- Precise movements, even in tight spaces
- Better access for complex cases

Jennifer shared:

Haley C. Horn

"The tiny incisions blew me away. I was expecting a big scar, but I only have a few faint marks. I was up and moving faster than I imagined."

Things to Keep in Mind

Limitations to Be Aware Of:
- Steep learning curve for surgeons
- Not available at all hospitals
- Higher upfront equipment costs
- Longer setup time
- Not suitable for every patient

Dr. Martinez often reminds patients:
"Technology is a tool, not the surgeon. The most advanced robot won't replace good surgical judgment."

Understanding the Cost Puzzle

Financial Factors:
- Robotics require expensive equipment, maintenance, and staff training
- Some insurance plans may limit coverage
- Out-of-pocket costs can vary widely

Questions to Ask:
1. Is robotic or laparoscopic surgery covered by my insurance?
2. Are there additional facility or equipment fees?
3. Will this option reduce recovery time, lowering indirect costs like missed work?

Haley C. Horn

Tip: Contact your insurance early for pre-authorization and cost estimates.

Choosing the Right Surgeon

Technology is only as good as the hands that use it.

What Makes a Great Minimally Invasive Surgeon?
- Performs a high number of laparoscopic or robotic cases yearly
- Has specialized training and certifications
- Low complication and conversion rates
- Explains the procedure clearly and patiently

Louis' story stands out:
"I spoke with three surgeons. The most tech-savvy one didn't feel right. The one who took the time to explain everything and even suggested a less expensive laparoscopic option earned my trust—and got me the best outcome."

Your Checklist for Surgeon Selection

- ☐ Case volume: More experience = better results
- ☐ Conversion rate : How often robotic/laparoscopic cases switch to open surgery
- ☐ Complication history : Honest discussion of possible risks
- ☐ Alternative approaches : Are you being offered the best option for YOU?

Haley C. Horn

- [ ] Emergency readiness : Does the hospital have backup plans?

Dr. Thompson advises:
"Choose the surgeon, not the robot. Their experience, judgment, and communication are what matter most."

While laparoscopic and robotic-assisted hysterectomies can make surgery feel less daunting, they are not miracle cures. The key is matching the right procedure to the right patient — and making sure your surgeon has the skills and experience to get you safely to the other side.

Hysterectomy Before Children: Navigating a Difficult Decision

Emma, a 32-year-old woman contemplating a hysterectomy due to severe adenomyosis, confided:
> "I always thought I'd be a mother."

This deeply personal statement highlights one of the most emotionally challenging aspects of hysterectomy — the impact on future fertility.

Emotional Considerations

Haley C. Horn

Choosing to undergo a hysterectomy before having children is a highly personal and difficult decision, often accompanied by a range of intense emotions.

Processing the Decision

Initial Grief and Shock

Learning that a hysterectomy may be the only medical option can feel overwhelming. Many experience a profound sense of loss — of future dreams, parenting hopes, or an envisioned life path.

- Acknowledging grief: Allow yourself time to mourn. Grieving is a normal and necessary part of making life-changing decisions. Journaling, therapy, or confiding in a trusted friend can help validate your emotions.
- Shock and disbelief: It's common to feel numb or struggle to accept the reality of the situation. Give yourself space and time to process the information before making decisions.

Fear of Regret

You may wonder if you'll regret your decision years from now — especially if you're unsure about parenthood or had hoped to have children someday.

- Seeking perspective: Connect with women who have faced similar choices. Support groups and online communities can offer valuable insights and

help you better understand the long-term emotional impact.
- Exploring alternatives: If preserving fertility is important, consult with a specialist about options such as egg or embryo freezing. Even if you ultimately proceed with hysterectomy, knowing you explored all possibilities can reduce future regret.

Identity Questions

For many, the ability to have biological children is tied to personal identity, femininity, or life purpose.

- Redefining womanhood: Remember, your worth is not defined by your reproductive capacity. Embrace the diverse aspects of who you are — your relationships, talents, and the contributions you make to the world.
- Reevaluating life goals: Parenthood takes many forms, including adoption, fostering, mentorship, or nurturing meaningful connections.

Relationship Concerns

You may worry about how this decision will affect your current or future relationships.

- Open communication: If you're partnered, have honest conversations about your feelings, concerns, and hopes. Reassure each other that you will face this challenge together.
- Future relationships: If you are single, it is normal to wonder how this might affect future partners. Remember, the right partner will respect and love

you for who you are, not solely for your reproductive potential.

Future Uncertainty

The prospect of life after hysterectomy may cause anxiety regarding hormonal changes, health, or emotional well-being.

- Empower through knowledge: Learn about the physical and emotional aspects of life post-hysterectomy. The more you understand, the less fearful you may feel.
- Build a support system: Lean on healthcare professionals, trusted friends, family, and communities who can offer guidance and emotional support.

Dr. Martinez, Reproductive Psychologist:
```
"The loss of fertility, even when medically
necessary, represents a significant life
transition that deserves acknowledgment and
support."
```

Stages of Acceptance

Accepting the decision may involve progressing through several emotional stages. These phases are not linear, and you may revisit them multiple times.

1. Shock and Denial

Haley C. Horn

Disbelief of Diagnosis

Receiving a recommendation for hysterectomy can feel surreal, especially if the condition was unexpected or symptoms were mild.

- What helps: Give yourself time to process. Ask your doctor detailed questions and don't hesitate to seek second consultations to clarify your understanding.

Seeking Multiple Opinions

It is common to search for alternative medical opinions in hopes of finding another option.

- What helps: While seeking opinions is valid, limit the number to avoid emotional exhaustion. Focus on guidance from trusted and qualified specialists.

Exploring Alternatives

You may instinctively look for less invasive options or temporary solutions.

- What helps: Thoroughly investigate all possible alternatives, including fertility preservation methods. Even if you proceed with hysterectomy, knowing you explored every option can provide peace of mind.

Emotional Numbness

Some people feel emotionally numb or disconnected as a coping mechanism.

- What helps: Recognize that numbness is often temporary. Therapy, journaling, or safe conversations can help you reconnect with your emotions.

Difficult Decision-Making
You may become paralyzed by the fear of making the "wrong" decision.

- What helps: Break down the decision into manageable steps. Weigh the pros and cons, seek advice from loved ones and professionals, and remember that you don't have to decide alone.

2. Anger and Grief

"Why Me?" Feelings
A deep sense of injustice is common.

- What causes this: Loss of control and altered future plans often fuel these emotions.
- What helps: Express your feelings through journaling or therapy. Self-compassion is essential — remind yourself that this situation is not your fault.

Mourning Future Dreams
Grief may focus on the loss of biological motherhood or an imagined family.

- What helps: Honor this grief. Consider alternative paths to parenthood such as adoption or fostering. Allow yourself space to reimagine your future.

Physical Symptoms
Grief often triggers physical symptoms like fatigue, headaches, or sleep disturbances.

- What helps: Prioritize self-care. Gentle activities, mindfulness, and adequate rest can help. Seek professional help if symptoms become overwhelming.

Emotional Outbursts
Anger may surface unexpectedly as frustration, irritation, or sadness.

- What helps: Find healthy outlets for anger, such as talking with someone you trust, physical exercise, or creative expression.

Relationship Strain
Miscommunication or differing coping styles can cause tension.

- What helps: Honest, open dialogue with loved ones helps. If needed, seek couples or family counseling.

3. Processing and Adjustment

Understanding the Options
Gaining knowledge often brings relief.

- Learn about the types of hysterectomy, recovery expectations, and potential long-term effects.
- Understand fertility preservation possibilities (egg or embryo freezing, surrogacy).

Exploring Alternatives
Make sure all options have been considered.

- What helps: Weigh alternatives such as medication, myomectomy, or other fertility-sparing procedures. Seek second or third opinions to ensure confidence in your choice.

Seeking Support
Support is vital during this period.

- Join online or in-person support groups.
- Express your feelings openly with loved ones.
- Therapy can provide a structured space for emotional processing.

Making Peace
Acceptance involves integrating this experience into your life without diminishing its significance.

- Re-examine your values and goals.
- Celebrate your resilience.
- Consider personal rituals or reflections to honor your journey.

Moving Forward

This phase involves embracing your new reality while honoring the challenges you've faced.

- Redefine your identity beyond biological parenthood.
- Set new short-term and long-term goals.
- Recognize your strength and adaptability.

| Rachel's Journey: |

Haley C. Horn

> "The toughest thing wasn't the surgery; it was accepting that my route to parenthood would be different than I had anticipated. Finding support allowed me to see different options."

Alternative Family Planning

For those facing hysterectomy before children, alternative family planning can offer hope.

1. Egg Freezing (Oocyte Cryopreservation)

A highly considered option if the ovaries are still functional.

Timing
- Egg quality and quantity decline with age, so early consultation is advised.
- The entire process takes around 2–6 weeks.

Cost Considerations
- Procedure costs range from $6,000 to $15,000 per cycle.
- Annual storage fees typically range from $500 to $1,000.
- IVF and surrogacy in the future may incur additional costs.

Success Rates
- Eggs frozen under the age of 35 have a higher chance of leading to a successful pregnancy.
- Clinics often aim to freeze 10–20 mature eggs for optimal chances.

- Live birth rates from frozen eggs range between 2–12%, depending on age and egg quality.

Storage Duration
- Eggs can be stored for many years thanks to advances in cryopreservation.

Future Usage
- Frozen eggs can later be used with IVF, possibly with a gestational carrier.
- Explore alternative parenting options like embryo freezing (if applicable) or adoption.
- Emotional preparation is equally important as logistical planning.

2. Surrogacy

Surrogacy offers a path to have a biological child through a gestational carrier, but it comes with legal, financial, emotional, and relationship considerations.

What is Surrogacy?
A gestational surrogate is a woman who carries a pregnancy for intended parents using embryos created via in vitro fertilization (IVF). This allows you to have a biological child, but it involves careful preparation.

Legal Considerations

Surrogacy laws vary significantly between countries and states. Legal guidance is essential to avoid complications.

- Surrogacy laws:
  - Some jurisdictions fully permit surrogacy, while others restrict or prohibit it.
  - In certain areas, intended parents may even need to legally adopt their biological child after birth.

- Contracts:
  - Legal agreements should outline the rights and responsibilities of all parties, including compensation, medical decisions, and parental rights.

- What to do:
  - Work with an experienced reproductive law attorney familiar with your region's laws.

Finding a Surrogate

Selecting the right surrogate is crucial.

- Agency Surrogacy:
  - Many use surrogacy agencies to match with qualified carriers who have passed medical and psychological screenings.
  - Agencies assist with logistics like doctor visits and legal matters.

- Independent Surrogacy:
  - Some prefer finding a surrogate from personal networks (friends or family).
  - This can be more affordable but requires careful legal and emotional navigation.

- Eligibility:
  - Surrogates should undergo health checks, psychological assessments, and fertility evaluations.
  - Establish clear boundaries and open communication early.

Financial Considerations

Surrogacy is a significant financial investment.

- Estimated Costs:
  - Typically ranges between $80,000–$200,000, covering agency fees, IVF, legal costs, surrogate compensation, and potential travel.

- Insurance:
  - IVF might be partially covered by insurance, but surrogacy itself is rarely included.

- What to do:
  - Research grants, loans, and fertility financing programs.
  - Plan for unexpected costs by building an emergency fund.

Emotional Readiness

Surrogacy is an emotional journey.

- Common feelings:
  - Grief, loss, or inadequacy due to the inability to carry a pregnancy.
  - Anxiety about entrusting someone else with your baby's development.

- Joy and excitement about becoming a parent.

- What helps:
  - Individual or couples counseling.
  - Open and honest communication with your surrogate.
  - Building a support network of family and friends.

Family Involvement

Surrogacy may also affect extended family dynamics.

- Educate loved ones:
  - Help them understand the surrogacy process and your reasons for choosing it.

- Family as surrogates:
  - Some family members may offer to carry the baby, strengthening bonds but requiring additional legal clarity.

- Support system:
  - Involve family as emotional and practical support during the process.

3. Adoption

Adoption provides another meaningful way to become a parent. Each form of adoption offers unique challenges, timelines, and financial considerations.

Types of Adoption

- Domestic Adoption:

- Adopting within your country through private or public agencies.
  - Can involve newborns or children waiting in foster care.

- International Adoption:
  - Adopting from another country, considering international laws, cultural factors, and immigration processes.

- Foster-to-Adopt:
  - Fostering a child with the possibility of adopting later.
  - Generally lower in cost but may come with legal uncertainty regarding permanent placement.

- Private Adoption:
  - Direct arrangement between birth and adoptive parents, often involving attorneys.
  - Offers more flexibility but may be costly.

Choosing an Adoption Agency

- What to look for:
  - Licensed and accredited organizations.
  - Agencies with successful adoption records and post-adoption support services.

- Questions to ask:
  - How are matches made between parents and children?
  - What are the estimated costs and timelines?
  - What level of openness (contact with birth parents) is expected?

- Tip:
  - Attend orientation sessions or seminars and speak with other adoptive families.

Home Study Process

A mandatory assessment to confirm you are prepared to adopt.

- Components:
  - Interviews, background checks, home inspection, and personal document reviews.

- Preparation:
  - Be transparent about your parenting philosophy and motivations.
  - Prepare your home to meet safety standards.

- Duration:
  - Typically takes 3–6 months.

4. Child-Free Living

Choosing a child-free life after a hysterectomy can be a conscious and empowering decision. Many find deep fulfillment by focusing on other meaningful goals.

Planning a Child-Free Life

- Financial freedom:

- Without the costs of raising children, you can prioritize wealth-building, early retirement, philanthropy, or travel.

- Lifestyle design:
  - Pursue hobbies, personal development, education, or entrepreneurship.
  - Plan for aging and long-term care without relying on children.

- What helps:
  - Create a clear personal life plan with evolving short- and long-term goals.

Navigating Relationships

- With your partner:
  - Discuss shared values and vision for the future.
  - Periodically revisit the decision to remain child-free as circumstances evolve.

- With family and friends:
  - Be prepared for questions or assumptions.
  - Set healthy boundaries while sharing your perspective confidently.

- What helps:
  - Counseling can support relationship dynamics.
  - Engage with communities or networks of other child-free individuals.

Finding Fulfillment

- Deepen connections:
  - Invest time in relationships, mentorships, or community engagement.

- Personal goals:
  - Explore travel, creative pursuits, volunteerism, or activism.

- Redefine legacy:
  - A legacy isn't limited to parenting. It can include the positive impact you make through your actions, work, or contributions to others.

- What helps:
  - Self-reflection, mindfulness, and professional guidance can help in finding meaning and joy on your unique path.

Time-Sensitive Decisions: Planning Before Surgery

If you are facing a hysterectomy and hope to preserve your fertility, early planning is key. While this process may feel overwhelming, knowing your options and working closely with healthcare professionals can help you make informed and empowered choices.

1. Fertility Consultation

- Why it matters: A fertility consultation gives you the opportunity to explore your options, learn what is feasible, and understand how fertility preservation can fit into your treatment timeline.
- What to expect:
  - You will meet with a reproductive endocrinologist who will review your medical history and assess your fertility potential.
  - Together, you will discuss preservation options, timelines, costs, and likely success rates.

Tip: The earlier you can have this conversation—even if you are unsure about wanting children—the more options you may have.

2. Hormone Testing

- Purpose: Hormone testing helps evaluate your ovarian reserve, giving you and your specialist a clearer picture of your current fertility status.
- Common tests:
  - AMH (Anti-Müllerian Hormone) — Gives an estimate of the number of eggs remaining.
  - FSH (Follicle-Stimulating Hormone) and Estradiol — Show how your ovaries are functioning.
- Good to know:
  - These are simple blood tests and results are typically available within a few days.
  - Results will help tailor your fertility preservation plan to your needs.

3. Egg Retrieval

- What it is: A process where mature eggs are collected from your ovaries and either frozen or fertilized to create embryos.
- Steps involved:
  1. Hormonal stimulation to help multiple eggs mature.
  2. Frequent monitoring with ultrasounds and blood tests to track egg growth.
  3. A minor outpatient procedure to retrieve the eggs using a thin needle under ultrasound guidance.
- Timing: The whole process typically takes 2–3 weeks, though individual timelines may vary.
- Things to keep in mind:
  - Not every retrieved egg may be suitable for freezing or fertilization, which is completely normal.
  - Success rates depend on age, ovarian reserve, and other health factors, but your fertility specialist will guide you through realistic expectations.

4. Embryo Creation

- What it involves: Fertilizing retrieved eggs with sperm to create embryos for future use.
- Considerations:
  - You can use sperm from a partner or a donor, depending on your situation.
  - You'll decide how many embryos to create, balancing emotional, financial, and practical factors.
- Why some choose this route: Embryos generally have higher success rates compared to freezing unfertilized eggs, but it's a deeply personal choice.
- Reassurance: You don't have to decide alone—your care team can walk you through the pros and cons.

5. Storage Arrangements

- How it works: After collection, your eggs or embryos are safely stored in a cryopreservation facility.
- Points to consider:
    - Storage fees typically range from $500 to $1,000 per year, with some clinics offering long-term plans.
    - Eggs and embryos can remain frozen for many years without losing viability.
- Important:
    - You'll likely be asked to complete legal forms about how you'd like your eggs or embryos handled in different scenarios, such as life changes or medical emergencies.
- Support: Many fertility clinics offer counseling to help you navigate these decisions thoughtfully.

Medical Considerations

As you consider fertility preservation, it's important to balance your hopes for the future with your current health situation. Understanding how your condition, treatment urgency, and recovery may influence your options will help you make the best possible choices with your care team.

1. Treatment Urgency

The urgency of your hysterectomy will significantly affect which fertility preservation options are available to you.

- If your surgery is planned (elective):

Haley C. Horn

  - You may have more time to complete fertility preservation steps such as egg or embryo freezing.
  - Your healthcare team can help you build a timeline that allows you to pursue these options without compromising your health.

- If your surgery is urgent:
  - In situations involving cancer, severe bleeding, or other emergencies, fertility preservation options may be more limited.
  - However, alternatives like ovarian tissue freezing—which can sometimes be done quickly or even during surgery—might still be considered.

- **Tip:** Always share your fertility goals openly with your medical team, even in urgent situations. They will help you find the safest and most realistic path forward.

2. Health Impact

Your underlying health plays a key role in determining what fertility preservation methods are safe and suitable.

- Existing conditions:
  - Health conditions such as cancer, severe endometriosis, or autoimmune disorders may limit certain options or influence the success rates of fertility preservation.
  - Some conditions may make hormone stimulation riskier, so your team will carefully assess if it's right for you.

- Hormone considerations:

- Fertility treatments often involve hormonal medications, which may temporarily impact your symptoms or interact with your existing condition.

- What you can do:
  - Be sure to give both your gynecologist and fertility specialist a full picture of your medical history, medications, and concerns.
  - Together, they will design a preservation plan tailored to your health and safety.

3. Recovery Time

Timing is everything, especially when balancing fertility preservation and the need for surgery.

- Egg retrieval recovery:
  - The egg retrieval process usually takes about 2–3 weeks, including hormone stimulation and monitoring.
  - Most people experience mild discomfort, bloating, or cramping for a few days afterward.

- Ovarian tissue freezing:
  - If time is especially limited, ovarian tissue freezing may be performed alongside your hysterectomy, helping reduce delays.

- Scheduling your hysterectomy:
  - In some cases, fertility preservation may slightly delay surgery.
  - Your healthcare team will help you decide whether a short delay is safe and appropriate for you.

Haley C. Horn

4. Success Rates

It's natural to wonder about your chances of successfully having a child later—and your specialist will help you understand this clearly and compassionately.

- Egg freezing:
    - Younger patients tend to have higher success rates, especially if eggs are frozen before age 35.
    - However, eggs can still be viable at older ages, depending on your ovarian reserve.

- Embryo freezing:
    - Embryos often have higher success rates than frozen eggs since fertilization has already occurred.

- Ovarian tissue freezing:
    - This method is still considered experimental in some places, and success rates can vary depending on your condition and the quality of the preserved tissue.

- Helpful mindset:
    - Your specialist will give you honest, personalized statistics and help you weigh the options with your unique health and goals in mind.

5. Future Implications

Beyond the immediate steps, fertility preservation has long-term considerations worth thinking through.

- Pregnancy options:
  - Without a uterus after hysterectomy, a gestational surrogate will be needed to carry a future pregnancy.
  - Surrogacy can be a fulfilling option, but it comes with legal, financial, and emotional factors.

- Health considerations:
  - Some fertility treatments could temporarily impact your health, especially if you have conditions like PCOS or cancer.
  - Your doctors will help minimize any risks while supporting your fertility goals.

- Emotional readiness:
  - Preserving fertility does not guarantee a future pregnancy. It's okay to have mixed feelings—many do.
  - Consider speaking with a fertility counselor to process emotions and expectations along the way.

- Legal and ethical factors:
  - Fertility preservation may involve legal decisions, especially when embryos are created.
  - Your care team may recommend a reproductive lawyer to help you make sure all paperwork is clear and protective of your wishes.

Financial Planning

While fertility preservation offers hope, it can also bring up questions about finances. Many people find this part of the process overwhelming, but you are not alone. With some research and guidance, you can make a financial plan that fits your situation and gives you more confidence moving forward.

1. Insurance Coverage

Your first step is to check if your health insurance offers any help with fertility preservation costs.

- Coverage for fertility preservation:
  - Some insurance plans cover part or all of the expenses, especially if your surgery is related to cancer or another serious medical condition.
  - Coverage might include consultations, hormone medications, egg retrieval, and embryo freezing.

- Local laws and mandates:
  - In certain regions, laws may require insurance companies to help cover fertility preservation when it is medically necessary.
  - Ask your doctor or a fertility clinic if such protections apply where you live.

- Helpful tip:
  - Call your insurance provider directly and ask for a detailed list of what's covered.
  - Try to get preauthorization for treatments if needed, so there are fewer surprises later.

2. Preservation Costs

Haley C. Horn

It's okay if fertility preservation costs feel like a lot to process—they often do. Knowing the general price range can help you plan step by step.

- Egg freezing:
  - Typically costs between $6,000 and $15,000 for the full process, including hormone stimulation, monitoring, and egg retrieval.
  - Annual storage fees range from $500 to $1,000.

- Embryo freezing:
  - Embryo creation adds fertilization costs, making the total between $8,000 and $20,000.
  - Like egg freezing, ongoing storage fees will apply.

- Ovarian tissue freezing:
  - Costs may range from $5,000 to $15,000 depending on your location and medical center.

- Medication costs:
  - Hormone medications used during stimulation can cost an additional $3,000 to $6,000.

- Tip:
  - Ask your fertility clinic for an itemized estimate so you can see exactly where costs come from.
  - Some clinics offer payment plans or partner with financial assistance programs to help make costs more manageable.

3. Future Treatment Costs

Fertility preservation is just the first step—down the road, you may also face costs related to using your frozen eggs or embryos.

- IVF (In Vitro Fertilization):
  - When you are ready to use your frozen eggs or embryos, IVF costs about $10,000 to $20,000 per cycle.
  - If additional procedures like genetic testing are recommended, this can increase the cost.

- Surrogacy:
  - Since you will need a gestational surrogate after hysterectomy, it's helpful to know that total surrogacy costs typically range from $50,000 to $150,000.
  - This includes surrogate compensation, medical care, and legal fees.

- Tip:
  - Don't be discouraged by these numbers. Many people find creative ways to plan, save, or access grants, especially when working with a fertility counselor or financial advisor familiar with these challenges.

4. Legal Expenses

Fertility preservation often involves legal considerations, especially when embryos, donors, or surrogacy are part of your plan.

- Embryo agreements:

- If you are creating embryos with a partner or donor, legal agreements will help define future use, ownership, and what happens in situations like divorce or death.

- Surrogacy contracts:
  - Surrogacy requires a legal contract to protect you, the surrogate, and the future child.

- Donor agreements:
  - If using donor sperm or eggs, legal guidance ensures a clear understanding of rights and responsibilities.

- Tip:
  - Consider setting aside $3,000 to $10,000 for legal fees, depending on your situation.
  - Look for a lawyer who specializes in reproductive law—they'll walk you through everything with care.

5. Long-Term Planning

Fertility preservation is a long-term commitment, not just financially but emotionally too. Taking a thoughtful approach now can ease the path ahead.

- Storage fees:
  - Keep in mind the ongoing cost of storing your eggs, embryos, or ovarian tissue, which could continue for years.

- Family-building timeline:
  - There's no rush, but it helps to think ahead about when and how you might want to start a family later on. Your

preserved eggs or embryos give you options, but not guarantees.

- Financial safety net:
  - Some people find it helpful to open a dedicated savings account, or use a health savings account (HSA) or flexible spending account (FSA) if available.

- Tip:
  - A financial advisor who understands reproductive health expenses can help you create a plan that balances fertility goals with other life priorities.

> Lisa's Reflection:
> "We had two weeks to decide about egg freezing before my surgery. It was overwhelming at the time, but I'm grateful we had the option and that my doctor and partner supported me every step of the way."

Practical Guidance

Making the decision to have a hysterectomy before having children can feel overwhelming. Practical tools can help you approach this process thoughtfully and with confidence. Whether you're just beginning to gather information or deep into decision-making, having a structured approach can reduce stress and bring clarity.

Decision-Making Tools

These tools can help you organize your thoughts, weigh your options, and make choices that align with your values and goals.

- Information Gathering
  - Learn about your medical diagnosis, treatment options, and potential alternatives.
  - Consult multiple specialists if possible, including fertility experts and mental health professionals.

- Timeline Creation
  - Outline a realistic timeline that balances medical urgency with emotional readiness.
  - Consider how much time you have to make decisions and what steps need to happen first (e.g., fertility preservation, counseling).

- Option Comparison
  - Compare the medical, emotional, financial, and personal impacts of different options, including surgery, fertility preservation, or alternative family-building methods.
  - Write down pros and cons to visualize your choices more clearly.

- Cost Analysis
  - Understand the financial implications of each choice, including fertility treatments, legal fees, and post-surgery care.
  - Explore available insurance coverage, grants, and financing options.

- Support System Building

- Identify people who can offer emotional, practical, or logistical support.
- Include friends, family, partners, healthcare providers, and support groups.

Questions to Consider

These questions may guide reflection and conversations with your loved ones or healthcare providers:

- How important is it to you to have biological children?
- What alternative family-building options feel acceptable or meaningful?
- What financial limitations or possibilities do you have?
- Who will be part of your support system during this journey?
- How much time do you have to make these decisions, medically and emotionally?

Professional Insight

> Dr. Thompson advises: "Take time to explore all options before surgery when possible. Even if preservation isn't chosen, knowing you considered everything helps with long-term peace of mind."

Reminders

- There is no one 'right' decision — only the one that is right for you.

- If you have time, allow yourself space to reflect before deciding.
- Seek out professional and peer support early.
- Consider documenting your process — journaling, audio notes, or creative outlets can help.
- Grief is a natural part of this process; allow yourself to feel it without judgment.
- Stay open to unexpected possibilities for fulfillment, family, or healing.

Talking to Your Doctor: Being Your Own Best Advocate

When I first started having symptoms, I didn't always share everything with my doctor. Sometimes I felt unsure, intimidated, or just eager to get through the appointment. Over time, I've learned that open, honest communication is one of the most powerful tools you have in navigating your health journey. Advocating for yourself doesn't mean being difficult — it means making sure your voice, questions, and feelings are heard and respected.

Helpful Questions to Ask

Good questions lead to good information. Here are some essential ones to help you feel more prepared when talking to your doctor:

About Your Condition
- What exactly is my diagnosis?

Haley C. Horn

- How severe is my condition?
- Is treatment urgent, or do I have time to consider options?
- What is the cause of this condition?
- Will it worsen without treatment?

About Treatment Options
- What are all the available treatment options?
- Why are you recommending this particular option?
- What would happen if I did nothing for now?
- What are the success rates and risks?
- How many of these procedures have you performed personally?

About Surgery Details
- What type of hysterectomy do you recommend and why?
- Will my ovaries be removed?
- What kind of anesthesia will be used?
- How long will the surgery take?
- What specific risks apply in my case?

About Recovery
- How long will I be in the hospital?
- When can I return to work or daily activities?
- What restrictions will I have?
- What signs of complications should I watch for?
- When will I be able to resume normal life activities?

Red Flags to Watch For

If you notice these signs, it may be time to seek a second opinion or look for a new provider:

- Your symptoms or concerns are dismissed or minimized.
- The doctor rushes through appointments.
- Alternatives to surgery aren't discussed.
- The doctor becomes defensive when you ask questions.
- Communication feels unclear or uncomfortable.
- The provider lacks sufficient experience with this procedure.
- You feel pressured to make a quick decision.
- They are unwilling to help navigate insurance issues.

Maria's Story:
```
> "When my doctor got irritated with my
questions, I knew it wasn't right. My
second-opinion doctor spent an hour patiently
explaining everything. That's when I knew I had
found the right surgeon."
```

Getting a Second Opinion

Seeking another perspective is normal — and often wise. You deserve to feel confident and informed.

When to Seek Another Opinion:
- Surgery is recommended as the only option.
- The diagnosis feels unclear or uncertain.
- You feel unsure about the proposed plan.
- You have a complex medical history.
- You want to explore all treatment options.
- Communication with your current doctor doesn't feel right.

How to Get a Second Opinion:

Haley C. Horn

1. Gather Your Records
   - Test results, imaging, lab reports, and treatment history.
   - Previous surgery or specialist reports.

2. Find Qualified Specialists
   - Ask for referrals.
   - Research credentials and patient reviews.
   - Confirm insurance coverage.

3. Prepare for the Appointment
   - Organize your medical history.
   - Make a list of current symptoms and medications.
   - Write down questions.
   - Bring a trusted support person.

How to Advocate for Yourself

You are your own best advocate. Here's how to stay empowered during your medical journey:

Know Your Rights:
- Access to all your medical records.
- Freedom to choose or refuse treatments.
- Full, informed consent.
- Privacy and confidentiality.
- Support navigating insurance.

Communicate Clearly:
- Be direct about your symptoms and how they affect your life.
- Keep a symptom diary to track patterns.
- Ask for clarification — no question is too small.
- Follow up if you don't understand something.

Build a Partnership:
- Share in decision-making whenever possible.
- Express your preferences and concerns.
- Ask for thorough explanations of all options.
- Maintain respectful communication, even when asking tough questions.

Dr. Thompson says:
> "The best patients are informed and engaged. Never hesitate to ask questions or seek a second opinion. It's your body, your choice."

What to Bring to Appointments

Having your documents ready helps you stay organized and confident.

Medical Records:
- Past surgeries and medical conditions.
- Allergies and medications.
- Family medical history.

Details of Your Current Condition:
- Timeline of symptoms.
- Past treatments and test results.
- Imaging and specialist reports.

Insurance Information:
- Coverage details and network providers.
- Pre-authorization requirements.
- Out-of-pocket costs and appeal processes.

Haley C. Horn

Legal Documents (if applicable):
- Advance directives.
- Health Care Proxy or Power of Attorney.
- Insurance cards and ID.

Lisa's Advice:
> "I made a binder with all my medical information. It was a lifesaver when meeting new doctors and dealing with insurance."

Appointment Tips

Before:
- Prepare questions in advance.
- Bring a friend or family member for support.
- Review your records ahead of time.
- Make sure you have transportation arranged.

During:
- Take notes or ask to record the conversation (with permission).
- Speak up about concerns or uncertainties.
- Confirm the next steps before leaving.

After:
- Review your notes.
- Follow up on pending questions or referrals.
- Update your medical file.
- Share important information with your support network.

Haley C. Horn

You deserve to feel heard and respected. Taking an active role in your care is not only allowed — it is essential. The right provider will welcome your questions and partner with you to make the best decisions for your health.

Choosing a Surgeon: Finding the Right Fit for You

Selecting a surgeon isn't just about qualifications — it's about trust, comfort, and partnership. After all, this is the person who will guide you through one of the most significant medical experiences of your life. You deserve someone who not only has the skills but also respects you, listens to you, and supports you.

When I was choosing my surgeon, I quickly realized that credentials alone weren't enough. I needed someone who understood my hopes, my fears, and my unique situation. You deserve the same.

What to Look for in a Surgeon

A great surgeon is more than technically skilled — they make you feel heard and cared for. Here's what to consider:

Haley C. Horn

Credentials & Experience:
- Board-certified in gynecology or gynecologic oncology (if needed).
- Specializes in hysterectomies or pelvic surgery.
- Has performed this procedure often — ask for specific numbers.
- Comfortable handling cases similar to yours.

Communication Style:
- Listens without rushing.
- Explains clearly in everyday language.
- Answer all your questions with patience.
- Welcomes your input and preferences.
- Respect your feelings, especially if you are navigating fertility concerns.

Supportive Office Environment:
- Friendly and helpful office staff.
- Good communication — prompt responses to calls and messages.
- Clear guidance about paperwork, scheduling, and insurance.

Emily's Reflection:
> "I knew I had the right surgeon when she said, 'I want you to fully understand all your options, not just the surgery.' She never made me feel like I was just another case."

Questions to Ask Potential Surgeons

Haley C. Horn

You don't have to be shy — you're allowed to "interview" your surgeon. Here are some helpful questions:

About Experience:
- How many hysterectomies have you performed?
- What type do you recommend for me, and why?
- What is your complication rate?

About Procedure:
- Will you perform the surgery yourself?
- What should I expect before, during, and after surgery?
- What are the risks and benefits specific to my case?

About Fertility and Hormonal Health:
- Will my ovaries be removed?
- What are my options if I want to preserve fertility or hormone function?
- Can I get a referral for fertility counseling if needed?

About Recovery:
- What is your approach to pain management?
- How long will recovery take?
- What follow-up care do you provide?

Second Opinions are Normal (and Smart)

Even if you like the first surgeon you meet, it's perfectly okay — and often wise — to get a second opinion. Different surgeons may recommend different approaches, especially if fertility preservation, medical conditions, or surgical techniques are involved.

Second opinions can give you peace of mind or reveal new options. The right surgeon will not be offended if you seek one.

Where to Find Potential Surgeons

- Referrals from your gynecologist or primary care doctor.
- Recommendations from trusted friends, family, or support groups.
- Research online — look for board certification, patient reviews, and hospital affiliations.
- Insurance network directories.

> Tip: If you are considering fertility preservation, you may want to consult with a reproductive endocrinologist alongside your surgical team.

The most important thing is that you feel comfortable and confident with your surgeon. You should never feel pressured, dismissed, or unheard. Trust your instincts — they matter.

Dr. Lee says:
```
> "Patients who feel informed and comfortable
with their surgical team tend to experience
less anxiety and have better recovery
experiences."
```

Helpful Reminders

- Take someone with you to consultations.
- Don't hesitate to write down your questions beforehand.

Haley C. Horn

- It's okay to take time before deciding.
- Trust that your feelings and concerns are valid.

Choosing a surgeon is a key step in your healing journey. You deserve a team that will walk alongside you with skill, compassion, and respect.

Anesthesia and You: Understanding Your Options and Feeling Safe

If you're feeling nervous about anesthesia, you are not alone. Many of us feel uneasy about "going under," but I promise — understanding what's happening behind the scenes can make a big difference. I used to worry about it myself, but once I learned about the process and met my anesthesia team, I felt much more at ease. Let's walk through what you need to know.

Types of Anesthesia for Hysterectomy

Most hysterectomies are done under general anesthesia, but there are other options in certain situations. Here's a simple breakdown:

General Anesthesia:
- You will be completely asleep and unaware during surgery.
- A breathing tube is used to support you safely.

Haley C. Horn

- Your vital signs (heart, lungs, blood pressure, etc.) are continuously monitored and controlled.
- This is the most common type used for hysterectomies.

Dr. Lee, anesthesiologist:
> "Think of general anesthesia like a carefully controlled 'pause button.' We are right there, every second, making sure your body is safe and comfortable."

Regional Anesthesia (Less Common):
- Includes spinal or epidural blocks.
- You remain awake but don't feel pain from the waist down.
- Occasionally used in specific situations, but not typical for hysterectomy.

Pre-Surgery Testing: Keeping You Safe

Your anesthesiology team will want to know everything about your health to create the safest plan for you. Expect these common pre-op tests:

Blood Tests:
- Check for anemia, bleeding risks, kidney and liver function, and blood type.

Heart Evaluation:
- May include an ECG (heart tracing) and blood pressure check, especially if you have heart risk factors.

Breathing Assessment:

- Checks lung function, sleep apnea history, and airway structure.

Full Medical Review:
- Your past surgeries.
- Current medications.
- Allergies.
- Family history of anesthesia problems.

Dealing with Anesthesia Anxiety

Many of us have common fears, such as:
- Will I wake up?
- What if I'm aware during surgery?
- How bad will I feel afterward?

You Can Ease These Fears:

1. Get Informed:
   Meet your anesthesiologist before surgery. Ask them to explain what will happen, how you'll be monitored, and how they handle any issues.

2. Practice Calming Techniques:
   - Deep breathing
   - Gentle meditation
   - Visualization
   - Listening to music
   - Asking about anxiety medication if needed

Annabel's Story:

Haley C. Horn
> "I couldn't sleep before surgery until I met
> the anesthesia team. They walked me through
> every step. It changed everything for me."

What Happens Right After Surgery?

In the First Hour:
- You'll slowly wake up in the recovery room.
- It's normal to feel a bit confused, sleepy, or chilly.
- Nurses will check your breathing, pain, and comfort closely.

In Recovery:
- You may have oxygen and IV fluids.
- Nurses will help manage nausea, pain, and any other symptoms.
- A support person will usually be updated while you're waking up.

Common Side Effects

Most side effects are temporary and manageable:
- Sore throat (from the breathing tube)
- Muscle aches
- Chills or shivering
- Nausea or vomiting
- Grogginess
- Temporary confusion or memory gaps

Your team is prepared with medications and care strategies to make you as comfortable as possible.

Haley C. Horn

Recovery Timeline After Anesthesia

- Day of Surgery: Grogginess, rest, limited awareness, frequent monitoring
- First 24 Hours: More alert, better pain control, starting to drink fluids, gentle walking
- Days 2-3: Clear thinking returns, less medication needed, back to regular meals, energy improving

Tips for a Smoother Recovery

Before Surgery:
- Follow fasting instructions.
- Get plenty of rest.
- Bring loose, comfortable clothing.
- Remove makeup, jewelry, and nail polish.
- Bring a trusted support person.

After Surgery:
- Take slow, deep breaths often.
- Move your legs gently in bed.
- Accept pain relief when offered.
- Stay hydrated.
- Don't hesitate to speak up if something feels off.

Dr. Thompson says:
> "Preparation and patience are the secret to a smooth anesthesia recovery. It takes time for your body to fully clear the medications — be kind to yourself."

The Good News,

Haley C. Horn

Anesthesia today is safer than ever, thanks to advanced monitoring and experienced teams. You are never alone in this — there is a whole team watching over you every step of the way.

Preparing for Surgery: Setting Yourself Up for a Smoother Recovery

Having been through a hysterectomy myself — and having helped many other women prepare — I can tell you that preparation is one of the best gifts you can give yourself before surgery. The more you set up in advance, the more you'll be able to focus on healing afterward. Let me walk you through how to get ready step-by-step.

Creating Your Healing Space at Home

You'll want to make your home a comfortable, safe place for recovery. Simple changes can make a huge difference.

Your Bedroom — Your Recovery Hub:
- Extra pillows (for propping and comfort)
- Side table stocked with essentials
- Phone charger within easy reach
- Adjustable lighting (think soft lamps)
- Entertainment (books, tablet, remote, headphones)
- Water bottle nearby

Your Bathroom:

- Raised toilet seat (if recommended)
- Non-slip bath mat
- Hand-held shower head
- Toiletries easy to reach
- Stool softeners ready
- Stocked toilet paper within arm's reach

Your Kitchen:
- Pre-made meals (freezer-friendly)
- Healthy snacks at waist level
- Paper plates and disposable utensils
- Step stool if you need to reach higher shelves
- Water stations throughout the house
- Consider arranging a meal delivery service for the first couple of weeks

Building Your Support System

Your Primary Caregiver (Week 1-2):
Having a trusted person nearby, especially during the first week, is essential.
- Help with personal care (showers, dressing)
- Medication tracking
- Meal prep and light housekeeping
- Transportation to follow-up appointments
- Grocery runs and errands

Your Extended Support Team:
- Meal train or food delivery help
- Childcare or pet care arrangements
- A friend for house cleaning or tidying up
- Someone to help pick up prescriptions
- Emergency contacts list ready

Haley C. Horn

Tip:
> A simple group chat or shared calendar can keep everyone on the same page and reduce stress for both you and your helpers.

Your Hospital Bag Checklist

Packing ahead will help you feel more settled the day of surgery.

Clothing:
- Loose nightgown or pajamas
- Robe
- Non-slip socks
- Front-opening sweater or cardigan
- Comfortable, loose going-home outfit
- Soft underwear

Personal Care:
- Lip balm (hospitals are dry!)
- Lotion
- Toothbrush & toothpaste
- Dry shampoo
- Face wipes
- Hair ties

Entertainment & Comfort:
- Phone & charger
- Tablet or e-reader
- Headphones
- Book or magazine
- Journal & pen

Haley C. Horn
- Small pillow for the car ride home
- Eye mask & ear plugs
- Family photos or a comforting item

Organizing Important Documents

Gather all paperwork in one folder or binder so it's ready when you need it.

Records:
- Insurance cards
- Medical history summary
- Medication list
- Allergy list
- Test results
- Doctor's instructions

Legal & Personal:
- Advance directive
- Health Care proxy
- Power of attorney (if applicable)
- Surgical consent forms
- Emergency contacts
- Pharmacy information
- Sick leave or disability paperwork

Financial:
- Insurance pre-approvals
- Payment plans (if needed)
- Budget for recovery expenses
- Any relevant FMLA or workplace forms

My Best Advice From Experience

When I look back, these things made the biggest difference:

1. Create Recovery Stations
   I had a small basket or table with essentials (snacks, medications, water, phone charger) in every room I spent time in.

2. Plan Your Support
   I made a clear schedule for friends and family so I wouldn't feel guilty asking for help. Everyone knew when and how to show up.

3. Simplify Your Home
   I moved frequently used items to easy-to-reach places and made sure my bedroom felt like a cozy healing nest.

Remember:
> It's okay to need help. Preparing ahead lets you focus fully on resting and healing when the time comes.

Getting Ready: Your To-Do List

Start preparing 2–3 weeks before surgery if possible:
- Review this checklist and adapt it to your space
- Communicate with your support team
- Practice using your adjusted home setup
- Pack your hospital bag early
- Organize and double-check documents
- Take deep breaths — you are doing a great job!

Haley C. Horn

The Day of Surgery — What Really Happens

I won't sugarcoat it — the morning of surgery is a swirl of nerves, hope, and vulnerability. I remember waking up, eyes wide open long before the alarm, wondering how I'd make it through. If you're anything like me, you probably wish someone would just walk you through what to expect, step by step, so you don't feel like you're free-falling. That's what I'm here for. Below is a gentle, honest guide to what most people experience on the day of their hysterectomy, from the first moments you open your eyes to when you wake up afterward.

Early Morning (4:30 – 5:00 AM) | At Home

This early part of the day feels strangely quiet — like the world hasn't woken up yet, but you have.

- Bathroom visit: Take a moment to empty your bladder before you leave home. It helps avoid unnecessary discomfort during check-in. If your surgeon asked you to do bowel prep the night before, you'll have already finished that part.

Haley C. Horn

- No food or drink: Hopefully, you stopped eating and drinking after midnight (unless your doctor gave you a specific exception). Having an empty stomach helps prevent anesthesia complications.
- Take only approved medications: If your doctor allowed certain medications (like blood pressure or thyroid pills), take them now with the smallest sip of water.
- Shower with special soap: Many hospitals give you antiseptic soap (often chlorhexidine) to lower your risk of infection. Wash well, especially around your belly, and skip lotions, perfumes, and deodorants afterward.
- Dress comfortably: Wear soft, loose clothes that won't irritate your abdomen later. I recommend easy slip-on shoes — bending over post-surgery is not your friend.

Early Morning (5:00 – 6:00 AM) | The Drive

This drive might feel surreal — like you're moving toward something huge but still in the quiet of pre-dawn.

- Leave early: Give yourself plenty of time. Hospitals usually want you there 1–2 hours before the scheduled surgery.
- Create calm: Play soft music, take deep breaths, or talk gently with your support person. You're allowed to feel nervous and hopeful at the same time.
- Mentally check in: Try a few grounding breaths. Inhale for four counts, hold for four, exhale for four. It won't make the fear vanish, but it will make space for calm.
- Double-check your essentials:
    - Photo ID
    - Insurance card

Haley C. Horn
  - Medication & allergy list
  - Advance directive or medical power of attorney (if you have one)
  - Comfortable clothes for after surgery

Arrival at the Hospital (6:00 AM)

This is where it starts to feel real — but also where things begin to feel a little more supported. You're not doing this alone.

- Check-in: You'll confirm your name, birthdate, and surgery details. They'll give you a wristband — wear it like a little reminder that everyone here knows who you are and why you're here.
- Meet your first nurses: They'll greet you, help you get settled, and walk you through everything ahead.

Pre-Op Prep (6:00 – 7:30 AM)

Now you're officially "in the system" for surgery, and the team will help prepare your body and mind.

Step 1: Changing
- You'll swap your clothes for a hospital gown, hairnet, and (often) compression socks.
- Remove jewelry, piercings, or anything that could interfere with surgery.
- A nurse will help store your belongings securely — or your support person can hold them.

Step 2: Health Checks
- Vitals: Blood pressure, heart rate, oxygen levels, and temperature — all routine.
- IV placement: A small IV will go into your arm or hand. This gives you fluids, meds, and later, anesthesia. It's a tiny pinch and then it's done.
- Pregnancy test: Even if you're sure you're not pregnant, this is standard for anyone of childbearing age.
- Final medical review: They'll ask you about medications, allergies, and your health history one last time.

Step 3: Meet Your Care Team
- Nurses: They'll stick with you throughout surgery and recovery. Don't be afraid to ask them anything — they're often the most comforting part of the process.
- Anesthesiologist: They'll explain how they'll keep you safely asleep and comfortable during surgery. Share any past reactions to anesthesia or concerns you have — nothing is too small.
- Your Surgeon: You'll have a final conversation, confirm the plan, and they'll likely mark your surgical site. This might feel formal, but it's actually a critical safety check.

Final Preparations (7:30 – 8:00 AM)

This part is like the final deep breath before the leap.

- Compression Devices:
  - Besides the compression socks, you'll likely get Sequential Compression Devices (SCDs) — soft wraps on your legs that gently inflate and deflate to keep your blood flowing during surgery.

- Catheter:
    - A Foley catheter will be placed to keep your bladder empty during surgery. This is often done after you've received some sedation, so it's usually not uncomfortable.
- Pre-Op Medications:
    - You might receive antibiotics, anti-nausea medication, and something to help you relax — all through your IV.
- Last bathroom trip: If you haven't had your catheter yet, this is your last chance. Nurses will help if you need it.

Before You Go Back

You'll get a few quiet moments where the surgical team does final checks and waits for the operating room to be ready. Some people cry. Some crack jokes. Some just breathe and stare at the ceiling. However you show up at this moment is okay.

When it's time, they'll wheel you toward the operating room. You might notice the cold air or the bright lights, but you won't be alone. Your anesthesiologist and nurses will be there, speaking calmly, making sure you're comfortable. Then, before you know it, you'll be asleep.

Mendoza's tip: "The hardest part for me was waiting. But as soon as I met my team and saw how calm they were, I started to believe I could do this too."

Haley C. Horn

The Operating Room — What Happens Once You're Inside

I want to gently prepare you for this next part because I remember feeling like I was stepping into the unknown. The operating room isn't like TV — it's less dramatic and more like a bright, organized workspace filled with people who know exactly what they're doing.

Entering the OR

- You'll roll into a room full of light and cool air.
- The OR team will be waiting — friendly, focused faces under surgical caps and masks. They're there just for you.
- You'll slide (with help) from the stretcher onto the narrow operating table. It's okay if it feels strange. They'll make sure you're safely positioned and comfortable.
- They may place heart monitor stickers (electrodes) on your chest and a clip on your finger to monitor your oxygen.
- The anesthesiologist or nurse anesthetist will talk you through what's happening and give you oxygen through a soft mask or nose tube.

Going to Sleep

This moment, while intimidating, is surprisingly gentle.

- You'll hear someone say something like, "We're giving you medicine to help you relax."

Haley C. Horn

- Within seconds of receiving the anesthesia through your IV, you'll start to feel drowsy.
- Most people remember hearing a few words or noticing the room fade — then nothing.

I promise, you don't need to do anything here. Your team will carry you through.

Waking Up — The Post-Anesthesia Care Unit (PACU)

This is where you'll wake up after surgery. And yes — you will wake up.

First Awareness

- The first thing you might notice is grogginess — like the deepest nap you've ever had.
- Nurses will be by your side checking your vitals, reassuring you that you're safe.
- You may hear someone calmly calling your name or asking you to take a deep breath.
- Expect a dry mouth, some abdominal discomfort, or even shivering — these are all normal, and the nurses are ready to help with all of it.

Pain Control

- One of the very first questions they'll ask is about your pain. Don't be shy — tell them the truth.
- Your IV will be your best friend here — they can give you pain medicine, nausea medicine, and fluids as needed.

- Some people feel very little pain right away, others more. Both are normal. The important thing is: your team is equipped to manage it.

The First Hours — Recovery Begins

After you're stable enough, you'll move from the PACU to your hospital room (or go home if you're having outpatient surgery).

In Your Room

- You'll still have the IV, catheter, and possibly SCDs on your legs.
- Nurses will continue checking your vital signs regularly — this is just routine.
- Your support person will likely be able to join you now, which brings comfort.
- You may feel tired, foggy, and a little overwhelmed. That's okay — you just did something monumental.

Pain, Nausea, and Mobility

- You might be surprised how quickly nurses will encourage you to start moving, even just sitting up or standing. Movement reduces your risk of complications like blood clots.
- Pain will be managed, but you'll still feel sore and tender — especially around your belly.
- You may notice gas pain in your shoulders or chest if you had laparoscopic surgery. It's harmless but uncomfortable. Walking helps!

Haley C. Horn

Your First Night

- You'll be closely monitored for pain, bleeding, and other routine post-op checks.
- Rest as much as you can, knowing that nurses are watching over you.
- Don't hesitate to ask for help — whether it's repositioning pillows, pain meds, or just someone to adjust your blanket.

Amelia's tip: "I thought waking up would be the scariest part, but honestly? It felt like waking from a deep sleep into the hands of people who knew exactly what to do."

Part 3: Returning to Movement and Life After Surgery

If you're like me, you might feel eager (and a little impatient) to get back to your usual rhythm after surgery. I want you to know that it's absolutely possible — but it takes patience, kindness toward yourself, and small, steady steps. Healing is not a race. It's a process, and you are allowed to move through it gently.

Safe Movement After Hysterectomy

The First 2 Weeks: Keep It Simple

- Walk Gently: Aim for short walks (5–10 minutes) around the house a couple of times a day.
- No Heavy Lifting: Nothing heavier than 5 pounds — think a bag of flour, not a full grocery haul.
- Daily Activities Only: Do only what's necessary (getting dressed, light cooking).
- Mind Your Posture: Good posture helps your core heal.
- Avoid Twisting: Move as a unit — no twisting at the waist just yet.

The Log Roll: Your New Best Friend

Haley C. Horn

The log roll technique helps you get in and out of bed safely, protecting your healing belly.

1. Roll to Your Side
   - Bend your knees.
   - Roll to your side, keeping shoulders, hips, and torso aligned.

2. Push with Your Arms
   - Use your arms to lift your upper body while letting your legs gently swing over the edge.

3. Move as One Piece
   - Avoid twisting. Keep everything moving together like you're rolling a log.

4. No Sit-Ups
   - Never try to sit straight up — it puts too much strain on your abdominal muscles.

5. Protect Your Core
   - Let your arms and legs do the work, not your healing belly.

> Why this matters: This technique helps you avoid injury, discomfort, or complications like hernias.

Tips to Make Log Rolling Easier

- Prepare Your Space: Add supportive pillows, and make sure your bed is at a good height.

- Move Slowly: No rushing. Gentle, steady movements win here.
- Ask for Help: It's okay to have someone assist you until you feel confident.
- Set Visual Reminders: Notes on your nightstand saying "Roll, don't sit up!" really help (trust me, I did this).

Sitting and Standing — The Safe Way

Getting up and down sounds simple — but after surgery, you'll need to be a little more thoughtful.

- Use Arm Supports: Press on armrests or sturdy furniture instead of pushing with your core.
- Neutral Spine: Sit and stand with your back straight but soft — no hunching or leaning forward too much.
- Gentle Core Engagement: Support your movement with a light brace of your abdominal muscles, without straining them.
- Take It Slow: Every movement can be deliberate. Slow is strong.
- Alternate Positions: Don't stay sitting or standing too long without changing positions.

> Why this matters: These habits protect your healing body, reduce pain, and make you feel more stable.

Graduated Movement Plan

You don't need to figure this out alone — here's a gentle guide to help you.

Weeks 2-4

- Walking:
    Start with 5-10 minutes twice daily. Slowly build up by adding 5 minutes every few days until you reach 20-30 minutes. Listen to your body and rest when needed.

- Gentle Movements:
    - Ankle pumps
    - Shoulder rolls
    - Pelvic tilts
    - Deep breathing
    - Supported stretches (avoid deep stretches)

Weeks 4-6

- Longer Walks
- Light Household Tasks
- Gentle Pelvic Floor Work (with guidance if possible)
- Balance & Body Awareness

Weeks 6-12

- Progressive Activities
    - Swimming (if your incision is fully healed)
    - Stationary cycling
    - Light resistance bands
    - Restorative or gentle yoga
    - Low-impact exercises

3-6 Months

- Return to Most Activities

- Gradual Strength Training
- Modified Core Work (avoid traditional sit-ups)
- Low-Impact Sports
- Progress at Your Own Pace

Listen to Your Body

Watch For:

- Increased pain
- Vaginal bleeding
- Fatigue
- Heavy pelvic or abdominal sensations
- Dizziness
- Shortness of breath

If you experience these, step back and rest. Adjust your activities and always communicate with your doctor.

Safe Core Alternatives

Instead of traditional ab exercises, try:

- Pelvic tilts
- Bridges
- Wall pushes
- Seated core work
- Standing balance exercises

> Dr. Thompson's advice: "If it hurts or makes you bleed, back off. It's not a failure — it's wisdom."

Returning to Work

Desk Jobs

- Most people return in 2–4 weeks.
- Start with shorter shifts if possible.
- Create an ergonomic workspace (good chair, proper desk height).
- Schedule regular movement breaks.

Physically Demanding Jobs

- Often requires 6–12 weeks depending on the nature of your work.
- A gradual return is key — lighter duties first.
- Open communication with your employer helps.
- Listen to your body daily and adjust as needed.

Success Tips for Returning to Work

- **Plan Ahead:** Talk to your supervisor about limitations and gradual return.
- **Support Counts:** Enlist coworkers or loved ones for help where possible.
- **Rest Without Guilt:** You are healing, not slacking.
- **Set Boundaries:** Protect your energy as you re-enter work life.

> Sarah's Story: "I returned to work half-days at first, and slowly built back up. My boss knew my limits, and I gave myself grace — it made all the difference."

- Progress is not a straight line — and that's okay.
- Healing takes time, but you are not alone in this.

Haley C. Horn

- Your body is doing something incredible — let it.
- If you feel stuck, scared, or unsure, reach out to your medical team or a pelvic health physical therapist.

Recovery Timeline

Looking back at my own recovery diary, I saw how each week brought new steps forward — sometimes big, sometimes small, but always meaningful. Knowing what to expect can help you move through your own recovery with more confidence and less fear. Here's a gentle, honest look at what the weeks ahead might hold.

Week 1: The Tender Beginning

This first week can feel overwhelming, but you are doing more than you realize simply by resting and breathing. Healing is happening, even when you feel still.

What to Expect:
- Pain Management is Priority
  Take your medications as prescribed — staying ahead of pain is easier than catching up to it. Ice packs, pillows, and short distractions (books, soothing sounds) can make a difference.

- Minimal Movement

Haley C. Horn

You'll mostly rest, with brief walks to the bathroom or around the room to prevent clots. Avoid lifting anything heavier than a full water bottle.

- Accepting Help
You'll likely need help with daily tasks — meals, standing up, personal care. This is normal. Receiving help is part of the healing, not a sign of weakness.

- Rest Without Guilt
Your only real job this week is to rest. Healing takes energy. Sleep often, nap when you can, and trust that this is productive.

- Tiny Victories Count
Sitting up unassisted? Walking to the bathroom solo? These moments are huge. Celebrate them — they are signs that you are already moving forward.

> My note from Week 1:
> ```
> "Today I walked to the bathroom alone. Small step for mankind, a giant leap for my recovery."
> ```

Week 2: Gathering Strength

This week is about gently expanding what you can do while still protecting your energy.

What to Expect:
- Easing Off Pain Meds

Haley C. Horn

You may start reducing prescription pain meds, possibly switching to over-the-counter options if approved. Some soreness lingers, but it should feel manageable.

- More Frequent Walks
Gentle walks — even a few loops around the house or yard — help your body and mood. Go slow, and rest when needed.

- Doing More, Bit by Bit
Dressing, bathing, preparing a simple snack — you might feel more independent now. But don't hesitate to still ask for help.

- Better Sleep
With pain easing, you may sleep more soundly. Supportive pillows remain your best friend.

- Healing on the Outside
The incision will likely be less swollen and less tender. But healing continues invisibly inside. Care for your scar gently and monitor for signs of infection.

Weeks 3–4: Steady Steps Forward

This is often the time when you begin to feel a shift — not fully back to normal, but noticeably better.

What to Expect:
- Light Activity Returns

You may feel ready for small tasks like folding laundry, light cooking, or watering plants. Keep avoiding anything that pulls on your abdomen.

- Driving (With Approval)
 If your doctor says you're ready and you're off narcotics, short drives may be okay. Prioritize safety — steering and braking need to feel comfortable.

- More Energy, but Fluctuating
 You'll have good days and tired days. Both are normal. Be gentle with yourself on the days you need more rest.

- Less Pain, More Awareness
 The ache may be dull, replaced by occasional twinges or pulling sensations. These are usually signs of healing tissues adjusting.

- Check-In
 You'll likely have a post-op appointment around now. Write down your questions ahead of time — they matter.

Weeks 5–6: Testing Your Wings

This is when many people feel ready to tiptoe back toward normalcy. The key is still: go slow.

What to Expect:
- Considering Work Return
 Many return to work in some capacity during this time. If possible, ease in gradually. Even desk work can be more tiring than expected.

- More Stamina
  Short walks may become longer. You might stay up later without crashing. Still, listen for the signs of "too much."

- Emotions May Surface
  This can be when the emotional impact of surgery shows up — relief, grief, frustration, or all of the above. You are not alone in feeling this way.

- Intimacy Talks
  Your doctor may clear you for sexual activity if healing is going well. Go at your own pace. Body changes may make things feel different — physically and emotionally.

- Gentle Exercise
  Light yoga, stretching, or swimming (if incisions are fully healed) may be okay. Avoid heavy lifting or core-straining moves.

Weeks 7–12: Finding Your New Normal

You're likely moving through life more freely now — but remember, you are still healing, inside and out.

What to Expect:
- Full Activity Returns (Mostly)
  Many resume work, social activities, and even low-impact exercise. Strength and endurance will continue to improve.

- Body Awareness

Some core weakness, fatigue, or twinges may still happen. Listen and respond — don't push through pain. Healing tissues may take up to a year.

- Emotional Shifts
You may still be processing the emotional layers of this experience. That's okay. Support groups, counseling, or simply talking it through with someone can help.

- Reclaiming Joy
As you feel more like yourself, hobbies, routines, and social connections become easier to enjoy again. Allow yourself this happiness — you've earned it.

- Scar & Body Care
Follow your surgeon's advice for scar care. And don't be surprised if your relationship with your body feels different. Be patient — your body has done something remarkable.

Each week holds its own challenges and victories.
You are not just recovering — you are adjusting, growing, and adapting. Healing is not linear, and neither is strength.

Be gentle. Be proud.

Understanding Your Post-Hysterectomy Body

Haley C. Horn

At my six-month mark, I thought I was finished healing. The incisions were closed, I felt stronger, and life seemed like it was returning to normal. Then came the surprises — little twinges, emotional shifts, waves of uncertainty I hadn't expected.

If you're here, you might be feeling the same. You're not alone. I've learned a lot through my own experience and through the hundreds of women who've shared their stories with me. Let's walk through what you might encounter — and what's worth paying attention to — as you adjust to your new normal.

What's Normal? What's Not?

Over time, your body will still speak to you — sometimes in familiar ways, sometimes with new sensations. Here's a helpful breakdown of what's common, and what signals a need to check in with your provider.

Normal Long-Term Experiences

These aren't signs of something wrong — they're common and often temporary.

Physical Sensations:
- Occasional twinges in the surgical area
- Weather-sensitive aches (yes, you might feel like a walking barometer)
- Temporary bloating

- Mild pelvic floor muscle spasms
- The sensation of scar tissue pulling as you move

Emotional Changes:
- Mood ups and downs
- Body image adjustments
- Shifts in identity
- Relief from chronic symptoms
- A new relationship with your body

> Rebecca shares: "Two years post-op, I still get occasional 'phantom cramps' around my period time. My doctor explained that this is normal — my body remembers its old rhythms."

When to Check In
If you notice these, don't hesitate to reach out to your doctor — you deserve peace of mind.

- Severe pelvic or abdominal pain
- Vaginal bleeding (after full healing)
- Fever or chills
- Difficulty with urination
- Persistent or worsening fatigue
- Depression or emotional distress
- Sexual discomfort or dysfunction
- Chronic, unrelenting pain

Hormone Changes — What You Might Notice

Haley C. Horn

Your experience will depend a lot on whether you kept your ovaries. Either way, hormone shifts are part of the landscape.

If You Kept Your Ovaries:
- Your body will still make hormones naturally.
- Menopause will come when it is always going to.
- Temporary hormonal fluctuations are common after surgery.
- Your ovaries may need occasional monitoring moving forward.

If You Had Your Ovaries Removed (Surgical Menopause):
Surgical menopause can feel like you suddenly flipped a switch:

Immediate Changes:
- Hot flashes and night sweats
- Mood swings
- Sleep disturbances
- Energy ups and downs

Long-Term Considerations:
- Bone health
- Heart health
- Sexual wellness
- Emotional balance
- Cognitive changes

```
> Dr. Thompson reminds us: "Think of hormone
changes like resetting your body's thermostat.
```

Eviction Notice

> It takes time to find a new normal, whether naturally or with support like hormone replacement."

Adjusting to Your New Body

Your body post-hysterectomy is still your body — but it might speak a new language.

Physical Adaptations

Core & Movement:
- You may need to modify exercise routines.
- Your pelvic floor might need attention (pelvic PT is amazing).
- You'll develop new patterns of movement and posture.

Body Signals:
- You might notice changes in weight distribution.
- Bladder and digestive patterns may shift slightly.
- Sexual response could feel different — but often improves with time and awareness.

> Maria shares: "It took me a year to fully understand my new body. Now I know its language better than ever."

Emotional Adaptations
Healing isn't just physical — it's also deeply emotional.

- Rebuilding trust with your body
- Integrating this surgery into your sense of self

Haley C. Horn
- Navigating changes in relationships
- Redefining self-image
- Gaining confidence

When to Call Your Doctor

Some signs are worth calling about, whether they show up early or long after surgery.

Urgent Symptoms:
- Sudden, severe pain
- Unusual discharge
- Fever over 100.4°F
- Trouble breathing
- Chest pain
- Swelling in one leg

Ongoing Concerns:
- Chronic pain
- Difficulties with intimacy
- Emotional struggles
- Bladder or bowel changes
- Extreme or persistent fatigue
- Any symptom that worries you

A Personal Look: Surprises Along the Way

Looking back, I wish someone had warned me about the hidden phases of recovery.

Month 3 — The "I'm Fine!" Phase:

- Feeling unstoppable
- Pushing past limits
- Ignoring small signals
- Forgetting you're still healing

Month 6 — The Reality Check:
- Unexpected fatigue
- Emotional waves
- Trust issues with your body
- Identity questions

Year 1 — Settling In:
- Learning to read your body again
- Accepting change
- Rebuilding confidence
- Knowing your limits and your strength

Year 2 & Beyond — True Integration:
- Feeling whole again
- Living comfortably in your body
- Emotional stability returning
- Adapting to this chapter of life fully

> Dr. Martinez gently reminds us: "Healing continues long after surgical scars fade. Physical and emotional adaptation is a process — and you are allowed to take your time."

Your body has changed, yes. But you haven't lost yourself — you're still here, learning, adapting, and reclaiming joy. Your new normal may be different, but it can be just as rich, deep, and fulfilling as what came before.

Part 4: Life After Hysterectomy

Hormone Replacement Therapy After Hysterectomy

When I woke up from surgery, one of the first things on my mind was hormones. Would I need them? What would happen next? Whether you've kept your ovaries or had them removed, understanding hormone replacement therapy (HRT) is an important part of caring for your body after a hysterectomy.

Types of Hormonal Changes

Your hormone journey after surgery depends on whether you kept your ovaries.

If You Kept Your Ovaries:
- Your body will continue producing hormones naturally.
- You likely won't need HRT right away — or at all.
- Your ovaries may still be affected by surgery stress, so mild fluctuations are common.

Haley C. Horn
- Regular monitoring is a good idea.
- Menopause may arrive slightly earlier than expected.

If You Had Your Ovaries Removed (Surgical Menopause):
This is a different experience entirely.
- Hormone production stops abruptly.
- Menopause symptoms tend to be more sudden and intense.
- The younger you are, the more important it is to talk about HRT.
- Your treatment plan should be tailored to your body, symptoms, and preferences.

> Dr. Roberts explains: "Without a uterus, you don't need progesterone to protect against endometrial cancer. This simplifies hormone therapy considerably."

Understanding HRT Options

If you and your doctor decide on HRT, there are multiple ways to tailor it to your life and needs.

Estrogen-Only Therapy:
Since your uterus is gone, you usually won't need progesterone — just estrogen.
- This simplifies dosing.
- Risk profiles are different from combination therapy.
- You have options to customize the dose and delivery method.

How You Can Take Estrogen

Eviction Notice 135

Haley C. Horn

1. Oral Tablets
- Easy to take daily
- Dosage adjustments are simple
- Widely available and affordable
- Good absorption
- Can be fine-tuned as you go

2. Transdermal Patches
- Applied twice weekly
- Provide steady hormone levels
- Avoid processing through the liver
- Gentler on digestion
- Convenient once you get the hang of it

3. Topical Gels or Creams
- Applied daily to skin
- Flexible dosing
- Absorbed directly
- Sometimes preferred for those with sensitive stomachs
- Can help with both systemic and local symptoms

4. Vaginal Estrogen Products
- Work well for vaginal dryness or discomfort
- Lower doses, localized effect
- Minimal absorption into the bloodstream
- Often used alongside or instead of systemic therapy

Making the Decision

Choosing HRT isn't just about symptom management — it's about improving your quality of life.

Haley C. Horn
Things to Consider:

Your Age:
- Under 45: Stronger recommendation to use HRT.
- 45–55: Depends on symptoms and risk factors.
- Over 55: Careful consideration with your provider.

Your Risk Factors:
- Family history (breast cancer, cardiovascular disease, blood clots)
- Bone density
- Lifestyle factors
- Personal medical history

Symptom Severity:
- Hot flashes
- Sleep disruption
- Mood changes
- Vaginal dryness
- Fatigue
- Changes in libido

Impact on Life:
- Work
- Relationships
- Emotional wellbeing
- Everyday activities

> *Sarah shares: "Starting HRT right after my ovary removal made the transition much smoother. I felt like myself again within weeks."*

Monitoring & Adjusting

HRT isn't a one-and-done situation. It often takes tweaks to get it right — and that's okay.

Typical Follow-Up:
- A check-in at around 3 months
- Annual reviews
- Adjustments based on how you're feeling
- Periodic tests depending on your risk factors

Tests to Consider:
- Bone density scans
- Cardiovascular screening
- Blood pressure and cholesterol checks
- Breast health exams

Common Adjustments You Might Need

- Changing your dose
- Trying a different delivery method
- Adding vaginal estrogen if needed
- Taking breaks if recommended
- Switching to non-hormonal options if HRT doesn't suit you

If HRT Isn't Right for You

Not everyone can or wants to use HRT — and that's okay too.

Alternative Options:

Natural Strategies:
- Nutrition tweaks
- Consistent movement
- Stress reduction
- Mind-body practices
- Good sleep hygiene

Non-Hormonal Medications:
- Certain antidepressants (SSRIs/SNRIs)
- Gabapentin
- Clonidine
- Some herbal supplements (discuss these with your doctor)

Situations Requiring Caution with HRT:
- Personal or family history of breast cancer
- Blood clot risks
- Significant liver or heart conditions
- Personal choice — you always get to say no

Dr. Cartier's Advice:
> "Start low, go slow, and listen to your body. Good HRT management is about patience and partnership with your care team."

Choosing whether or not to use HRT is personal — and there's no one-size-fits-all answer.

This is about you, your symptoms, your risks, and your quality of life.

Haley C. Horn

Your care team is there to help you find what works best, and it's okay if it takes a little trial and error.

SEXUALITY AND INTIMACY AFTER HYSTERECTOMY

When I sat in my support group six months after my hysterectomy, I noticed something: the most common questions weren't about pain or recovery — they were about intimacy. Will sex feel different? Will I enjoy it again? How do I even start?

These are tender, important questions. Let's have a gentle and honest conversation about intimacy after hysterectomy — the challenges, the surprises, and the possibilities.

Understanding Physical Changes and Adjustments

The initial healing phase after a hysterectomy is about more than stitches and scar tissue — it's about giving your body the care and patience it deserves. Knowing what to expect can help you move through this time with less worry and more confidence.

The Healing Window (First 6–8 Weeks)

1. Complete Pelvic Rest

- Pelvic rest usually lasts about 6–8 weeks and means avoiding sexual intercourse, tampons, and douching.
- This pause gives your body the best chance for smooth healing and helps prevent complications like infection or delayed tissue repair.

2. Ongoing Internal Healing
- Even after the external incisions have healed, internal tissues continue mending.
- Mild soreness, sensitivity, or cramping is common and usually improves over time.

3. Vaginal Changes
- If your cervix was removed, your vaginal length may be slightly shorter — but most people adjust without lasting discomfort.
- Hormonal shifts may cause vaginal dryness, which is common but very manageable with lubricants, moisturizers, or hormone therapies.
- Over time, vaginal tissues tend to regain elasticity and adaptability.

4. Hormonal Considerations
- If your ovaries were removed, you may experience a sudden drop in estrogen, which can affect libido, lubrication, and mood.
- Hormone replacement therapy (HRT) or non-hormonal options can help — this is a conversation worth having with your doctor.

5. Scar Tissue

- It's normal for some scar tissue to form internally. For some, this is barely noticeable, while others might feel slight tightness or tenderness.
- Pelvic floor exercises can gently stretch and strengthen muscles to reduce discomfort.

Gentle Tips for Early Healing
- Be patient — truly. Your body is working hard, even if you can't see it.
- Keep checking in with your doctor during follow-ups.
- Address vaginal dryness early if needed — there's no need to "push through" discomfort.
- Maintain open communication with your partner. There are many ways to share intimacy beyond intercourse while you heal.

What Might Feel Different — And Why That's Okay

For many, intimacy after hysterectomy feels different at first — but different doesn't mean bad. It simply means discovering your new normal.

1. Sensations May Change
- Some women notice changes in sensitivity, especially if the cervix was removed.
- Scar tissue may make things feel tighter or slightly uncomfortable at first.
- It can take months for nerves to fully heal — so allow your body all the time it needs.

> Tip: Begin with gentle, non-penetrative intimacy and explore slowly.

2. Lubrication Patterns Might Shift
- Hormonal changes (or simply healing) may reduce natural lubrication.
- Even if your ovaries remain, some women experience dryness after surgery.

> Tip: Use lubricants and moisturizers liberally and without hesitation — they're part of caring for your body, not a sign that something is wrong.

3. Finding What Feels Good
- After surgery, certain positions may feel better than others.
- Positions that reduce pressure on the pelvis or abdomen can be more comfortable.

> Tip: Side-lying or elevated positions are often helpful, and using pillows can make a big difference.

4. Discovering New Sensitivities
- Some people find that without the uterus or cervix, other areas — like the breasts, neck, thighs, or ears — become more responsive.
- The absence of uterine contractions during orgasm may shift where and how pleasure is felt.

> Tip: This can be an opportunity for exploration and creativity — intimacy is more than just mechanics.

5. Arousal May Take More Time
- It's common to need a longer warm-up, physically and emotionally.

Haley C. Horn

- Body image changes or emotional stress from surgery can affect desire.

> Tip: Prioritize connection and foreplay, and be kind to yourself if your arousal patterns have shifted.

Maria shares:
> "At first, everything felt different. But with patience and communication, my partner and I discovered that different didn't mean worse — just new."

Practical Ways to Enhance Intimacy

Reconnecting with your body — and your partner — may require some creativity and flexibility. Here are gentle, practical strategies:

1. Lubrication is Your Friend
- Use water-based or silicone-based lubricants generously.
- Try vaginal moisturizers regularly for ongoing hydration.
- If needed, ask about vaginal estrogen creams or HRT.

2. Comfort First
- Use positions that feel good to your body — comfort is key.
- Support your body with pillows and take your time.
- There is no rush; intimacy has no deadline.

3. Choose the Right Timing
- Pick moments when you feel rested and relaxed.

Haley C. Horn

- Listen to your body and honor its signals.

4. Relaxation Techniques
- Deep breathing, gentle movement, warm baths, and soft music can help ease tension.
- Intimacy thrives when the body feels safe and calm.

5. Pelvic Floor Care
- Pelvic floor exercises, guided by a physical therapist if needed, can help with flexibility, strength, and sensation.

Dr. Thompson reminds us:
> "Sexual health is part of your overall well being. Please don't hesitate to bring these concerns to your healthcare provider — they are here to help."

When Intimacy Feels Painful

If intimacy brings discomfort, you are not alone — and there are many ways to find relief.

Common Causes
- Internal healing and scar tissue
- Vaginal dryness
- Pelvic floor muscle tension
- Nerve sensitivity
- Emotional tension or anxiety

Helpful Solutions
- Start gently, with non-penetrative intimacy
- Use plenty of lubrication

- Explore positions that you control
- Consider pelvic floor therapy
- Keep honest, open conversations with your partner

When Extra Support is Helpful
- Persistent or worsening pain
- Bleeding or sharp discomfort during intimacy
- Overwhelming emotional distress about intimacy

If any of these arise, please speak to your healthcare provider. They want to help you feel comfortable and confident again.

There is no "right" way to experience intimacy after hysterectomy — only your way. For many, intimacy after surgery eventually feels just as good, or even better, than before. For others, it may take time and adjustment.

With patience, creativity, and communication, you can rediscover pleasure and closeness, honoring your body as it is now.

Pelvic Floor Health: The Unsung Hero of Recovery

Before my hysterectomy, I had no idea how much my pelvic floor did for me. It wasn't until after surgery, when I began noticing subtle shifts—bladder leaks, lower back aches, and intimacy feeling "off"—that I realized this quiet group of muscles was carrying more than I gave it credit for. If you're reading this, you might be noticing some of the same things. The good news? You're not powerless, and you're not alone.

With some simple knowledge and gentle effort, you can strengthen your pelvic floor and help it support you, not just in recovery, but for the rest of your life.

Your Pelvic Floor: Quietly Holding Everything Together

Think of your pelvic floor like a soft but reliable hammock stretched across the bottom of your pelvis. It's made of muscles, ligaments, and connective tissue, and its job is pretty incredible—it holds up your bladder, bowel, uterus (if still present), and supports your spine and core. It also plays a big role in how you feel during intimacy, how you control your bladder and bowel, and even how steady and strong you feel when you move.

After hysterectomy, your pelvic floor has to adapt. With the uterus gone, the whole system adjusts. That's why giving it some attention now is a powerful act of care.

How Hysterectomy Affects Your Pelvic Floor

Shift #1: A Change in Support

The uterus was part of your pelvic support system. Without it, your pelvic muscles and ligaments have to pick up the slack. For some, this shift can lead to things like pelvic organ prolapse (when the bladder, bowel, or vaginal walls begin to descend). It sounds scary, but with early awareness, you can help prevent or manage this.

What helps:

- Learn gentle pelvic floor exercises (we'll get to those soon).
- Avoid heavy lifting during recovery.

Shift #2: Pressure in New Places

Without the uterus helping absorb intra-abdominal pressure, your pelvic floor takes on more of the load. Coughing, laughing, sneezing, or lifting can feel different or trigger leaks.

What helps:

- Learn the "Knack": Gently contract your pelvic floor just before you cough, sneeze, or lift.
- Practice relaxed, belly-deep breathing to avoid pushing down on your pelvic floor.

Shift #3: Muscle & Nerve Changes

Surgery can leave pelvic muscles feeling weak, tense, or disconnected. Nerves may have been stretched or irritated. This can affect coordination, sensation, and control.

What helps:

Haley C. Horn

- Work with a pelvic floor physical therapist if you can—they are life-changing.
- Try biofeedback tools to rebuild your muscle connection.

Shift #4: Healing Takes Time

After surgery, scar tissue forms and muscles adapt. Movements that once felt automatic—getting out of bed, standing up, even sitting comfortably—might now require mindfulness.

What helps:

- Use the "log roll" method to get in and out of bed.
- Gentle stretching and pelvic tilts help blood flow and flexibility.

Shift #5: New Awareness

Many of us only start noticing our pelvic floor when something feels off—but this is actually an opportunity. Awareness is the first step to empowerment.

What helps:

- Keep a journal of symptoms and improvements.
- Don't hesitate to bring concerns to your doctor or pelvic floor specialist.

> Sarah's Story: "Once I started paying attention to my pelvic floor, I felt like I got part of myself back. It's about more than

```
avoiding leaks—it's about standing tall and
feeling strong again."
```

Gentle Exercises to Support Your Recovery

Step 1: Finding Your Pelvic Floor

The pelvic floor muscles are the ones you'd use to stop the flow of urine or hold in gas.

How to find them:

- During urination, try briefly stopping the stream. The muscles you feel? That's them. (Don't make this a habit, just a one-time identification.)
- Or imagine gently lifting the space between your sit bones, as if drawing something up inside you.

Step 2: Basic Pelvic Floor Contractions (Kegels)

Technique:

- Get comfy—lying down is a great place to start.
- Gently squeeze and lift the pelvic floor (like picking up a blueberry with your muscles).
- Hold for 3–5 seconds.
- Release fully, feeling a soft drop.
- Breathe throughout—no breath-holding.

Repeat 10 times, 2–3 times a day.

Haley C. Horn

Tip: Don't overdo it. More is not better—balance contraction with relaxation.

Step 3: Building Strength and Control

Once you're comfortable with basic contractions, you can gently progress.

- Quick flicks: Quickly contract and release 10 times.
- Endurance holds: Hold for up to 10 seconds if comfortable.
- Functional practice: Squeeze gently before coughing, laughing, or lifting.
- Integrate: Engage lightly while walking or standing for improved posture and stability.

Step 4: Working With a Specialist (If You Can)

Pelvic floor physical therapists are worth their weight in gold. They can teach you to:

- Coordinate your pelvic floor with breathing.
- Avoid common mistakes (like clenching your glutes instead).
- Rebuild strength, sensation, and confidence.

> Dr. Roberts, Pelvic PT: "Your pelvic floor is like a hammock that's been remodeled. It needs care, but it's more than capable of supporting you beautifully."

Haley C. Horn

Pelvic floor recovery is a journey, not a race. It's normal to feel awkward at first. It's normal to feel frustrated some days. But every gentle squeeze, every mindful breath, is helping your body trust you again.

Your pelvic floor isn't just about preventing leaks or prolapse. It's about feeling supported, comfortable, and connected to your body again — in all the ways that matter most.

> "Learning to properly engage my pelvic floor changed everything. It wasn't just about Kegels—it was about understanding my body's new normal." — Ava

Haley C. Horn

Glossary of Terms

Abdominal Hysterectomy
A surgical procedure to remove the uterus through an incision in the abdomen.

Adhesions
Bands of scar tissue that can form after surgery, causing tissues and organs to stick together.

Bladder
The organ that stores urine. Its position and support may be affected after a hysterectomy.

Bladder Training
A technique to improve bladder control by gradually increasing the time between bathroom visits.

Bowel
The intestines, responsible for digesting food and eliminating waste. Pelvic surgery may affect bowel function.

Cervix
The lower, narrow part of the uterus that connects to the vagina. It may or may not be removed during a hysterectomy.

Core Muscles

Muscles of the abdomen, back, and pelvic floor that work together to stabilize the spine and pelvis.

Diaphragmatic Breathing
A breathing technique that engages the diaphragm, promoting relaxation and helping to manage intra-abdominal pressure.

Dyspareunia
Painful intercourse, which can sometimes occur after hysterectomy due to pelvic floor dysfunction or vaginal changes.

Endometriosis
A condition where tissue similar to the uterine lining grows outside the uterus, often causing pain and infertility.

Estrogen
A hormone primarily produced by the ovaries, important for regulating menstruation, bone health, and vaginal tissue health.

Hysterectomy
The surgical removal of the uterus. It can be partial, total, or radical, depending on which structures are removed.

Hysterectomy Types
- Partial: Removal of the uterus, leaving the cervix intact.
- Total: Removal of the uterus and cervix.
- Radical: Removal of the uterus, cervix, part of the vagina, and surrounding tissues (typically for cancer).
- Supracervical: Another term for partial hysterectomy.

Haley C. Horn

Incontinence
The involuntary loss of urine or stool. It may be stress-related (due to pressure) or urge-related (sudden, intense need to go).

Intra-abdominal Pressure
The pressure within the abdominal cavity increases during actions like lifting, sneezing, or coughing.

Kegel Exercises
Pelvic floor muscle exercises that help strengthen and improve control of the muscles supporting the bladder, bowel, and sexual function.

Knack Maneuver
A technique of contracting the pelvic floor muscles before coughing, sneezing, or lifting to prevent urine leakage.

Laparoscopic Hysterectomy
A minimally invasive surgery to remove the uterus using small incisions and a camera (laparoscope).

Ligaments
Bands of connective tissue that help stabilize organs. Pelvic ligaments may need to be compensated after hysterectomy.

Log Roll Technique
A method of getting in and out of bed without straining the abdomen by rolling onto your side first.

Menopause

The natural or surgical cessation of menstruation, marked by decreased estrogen levels.

Oophorectomy
Surgical removal of one or both ovaries. If both are removed, it causes surgical menopause.

Ovaries
Organs that produce eggs and hormones (estrogen and progesterone). They may or may not be removed during hysterectomy.

Pelvic Floor
A group of muscles, ligaments, and connective tissue at the base of the pelvis that supports the bladder, uterus, bowel, and vagina.

Pelvic Floor Dysfunction
Weakness, tightness, or poor coordination of pelvic floor muscles, leading to symptoms such as incontinence, pelvic pain, or prolapse.

Pelvic Floor Physical Therapist
A specialist trained to assess and treat pelvic floor dysfunction using exercises, manual therapy, and education.

Pelvic Organ Prolapse
The descent of pelvic organs (bladder, rectum, or vaginal walls) into or outside of the vaginal canal due to weakened support structures.

Perimenopause
The transitional period before menopause when hormonal changes cause symptoms like irregular periods or hot flashes.

Haley C. Horn

Peritoneum
A thin tissue lining the abdominal cavity and covering pelvic organs. It is sometimes involved in surgical recovery.

Progesterone
A hormone produced mainly by the ovaries, important for regulating the menstrual cycle and pregnancy.

Rectum
The lower part of the large intestine leading to the anus. Its position may be influenced by changes in pelvic support.

Scar Tissue
Fibrous tissue that forms as part of the body's healing process after surgery, which can sometimes lead to discomfort or adhesions.

Stress Urinary Incontinence (SUI)
Leakage of urine due to pressure on the bladder from activities like coughing, sneezing, or lifting.

Surgical Menopause
Menopause caused by the removal of both ovaries, leading to an abrupt drop in estrogen.

Urethra
The tube through which urine exits the body. Its function can be affected by pelvic floor changes.

Uterus

Haley C. Horn

A muscular organ where a baby grows during pregnancy. Its removal is the core component of hysterectomy.

Vagina
The muscular canal leading from the cervix to the external genitalia. Vaginal length and elasticity may change after surgery.

Vaginal Hysterectomy
A surgical technique where the uterus is removed through the vagina without external incisions.

Vaginal Vault
The upper part of the vaginal canal after the removal of the uterus.

Vaginal Vault Prolapse
A condition where the top of the vagina descends after hysterectomy due to weakened support.

Vaginal Atrophy
Thinning and drying of vaginal tissues, often related to lower estrogen levels after menopause or hysterectomy.

Made in the USA
Middletown, DE
12 April 2025

74177692R00089